7-DAY
APPLE CIDER
VINEGAR
CLEANSE

7-DAY
APPLE CIDER
VINEGAR
CLEANSE

Lose Up to 15 Pounds in 7 Days and

Turn Your Body into a Fat-Burning Machine

JJ SMITH

SIMON & SCHUSTER PAPERBACKS

NEW YORK   LONDON   TORONTO   SYDNEY   NEW DELHI

Simon & Schuster Paperbacks
An Imprint of Simon & Schuster, Inc.
1230 Avenue of the Americas
New York, NY 10020

First Simon & Schuster trade paperback edition December 2019

SIMON & SCHUSTER PAPERBACKS and colophon are trademarks of Simon & Schuster, Inc.

For information about special discounts for bulk purchases, please contact Simon & Schuster Special Sales at 1-866-506-1949 or business@simonandschuster.com.

The Simon & Schuster Speakers Bureau can bring authors to your live event. For more information or to book an event, contact the Simon & Schuster Speakers Bureau at 1-866-248-3049 or visit our website at www.simonspeakers.com.

Interior design by Kyoko Watanabe

Manufactured in the United States of America

1   3   5   7   9   10   8   6   4   2

Library of Congress Cataloging-in-Publication Data
Names: Smith, J. J. (Jennifer J.), author.
Title: 7-day apple cider vinegar cleanse : lose up to 15 pounds in 7 days and turn your body into a fat-burning machine / JJ Smith.
Other titles: Seven day apple cider vinegar cleanse
Description: New York, NY : Atria Paperback, an imprint of Simon & Schuster, 2019. | Summary: "JJ Smith, author of the #1 New York Times bestseller 10-Day Green Smoothie Cleanse, provides an all-new and accessible detox system that rids the body of unwanted fat and bacteria for renewed energy and lasting weight loss. In the tradition of certified weight loss expert and nutritionist JJ Smith's 10-Day Green Smoothie Cleanse, Think Yourself Thin, and Green Smoothies for Life, comes the 7-Day Apple Cider Vinegar Cleanse. This revolutionary cleanse includes meals and drinks that help support the body's natural detoxification process and promote a healthy environment for good bacteria in the body. All of the new and delicious 25 recipes for breakfast, lunch, dinner, and snacks will effectively help rid of your body of toxins and unwanted fat in just 7 days, jump starting your journey to permanent weight loss"—Provided by publisher.
Identifiers: LCCN 2019031341 | ISBN 9781982118075 (paperback) | ISBN 9781982118082 (ebook)
Subjects: LCSH: Detoxification (Health) | Reducing diets—Recipes. | Cider vinegar. | LCGFT: Cookbooks.
Classification: LCC RA784.5 .S6435 2019 | DDC 613.2/5—dc23
LC record available at https://lccn.loc.gov/2019031341

ISBN 978-1-9821-1807-5
ISBN 978-1-9821-1808-2 (ebook)

Contents

Contents

7-DAY
APPLE CIDER
VINEGAR
CLEANSE

Introduction

Apple cider vinegar (ACV) has gained popularity for its multitude of health benefits. It has long been used as a home remedy, but in recent years ACV has gained traction for its ability to support weight loss, reduce cholesterol, lower blood sugar levels, and improve symptoms of diabetes. It can also be used for various household and cooking purposes.

For three years, I've taught the benefits of apple cider vinegar for detox and weight loss. My Apple Cider Vinegar Cleanse Drink was featured on *The Dr. Oz Show* and has been written about in *Woman's World* magazine. Dr. Oz said, "JJ Smith put ACV on the map and had eighteen million people follow her ACV detox drink video." Although apple cider vinegar has been around for centuries, it's awesome to be acknowledged for the impact I've had on increasing the popularity of this health tonic.

In fact, several ACV manufacturers have reached out to develop a partnership because they believe I have helped to boost the sales of their product. They are also experiencing customer growth and increased positive reviews, which they have attributed to my videos on ACV.

ACV has been used by my followers with great success, evidenced by the enthusiastic testimonials I have received. With that in mind, I've created a new cleanse that takes advantage of the health and healing properties of apple cider vinegar to help you take back control of your health and shed up to fifteen pounds in just seven days.

The 7-Day Apple Cider Vinegar Cleanse turns your body into a fat-burning machine. With the tools provided in this book, you will learn to melt away body fat in the shortest possible time. Our first goal is fast, healthy weight loss. Our second goal is to change how your body stores fat so that it will be harder for you to gain the weight back. Our third goal is to help you lay the foundation for living a longer, healthier life. The strategies that follow will help you keep your body in fat-burning mode so that permanent weight loss is no longer a struggle.

Some of the concepts taught in this book have been around for decades. I've put together a seven-day regimen that teaches you the secrets to burning fat faster while also reversing many health conditions. I like to simplify the complicated and conflicting information on weight loss so that you attain the success you desire, whether it's shedding a few pounds or the many that have made you obese. I am hoping that you follow this program right away so you and your family do not have to experience any obesity diagnosis. It's time to take control of your health and your weight.

I want to make two points about diets. First, when you follow any weight-loss plan or popular diet, you will lose weight right away. This is primarily because you are eating less food, usually less carbohydrates (carbs) and sugar. This causes you to have fewer insulin spikes, leading to reduced fat storage in the body. With excess insulin present, you cannot lose body fat. All diets follow this basic concept of eating less carbs and sugar. Second, you cannot lose weight and body fat simply by counting calories. Yes, calories are important. However, the number of calories you consume is not as important as the *type* of calories when determining how much weight you lose and how healthy you are.

How It All Started

A few years ago, after years of clean, healthy eating and detoxing, I became terribly ill. I was bedridden. It turned out I had gotten mercury poisoning from my silver dental fillings! There were high levels of mercury in my brain, gut, liver, and kidneys. I couldn't get out of bed for two months. When I did, just making the bed required that I lie back down to rest! My health, energy, and motivation were at an all-time low.

After a long and slow recovery, I decided I needed to do something to get my health and energy back as well as lose the twenty pounds I had gained while bedridden. After learning how raw greens can heal the body, I created my 10-Day Green Smoothie Cleanse. Already an advocate of detoxing, I knew I needed to rid my body of the waste and toxins that had accumulated as a result of the mercury poisoning.

As I wrote in my introduction to the *10-Day Green Smoothie Cleanse*, once I created that cleanse, I asked my community of friends and family if they would join and support me. My goal was to get ten people to say yes. I was pleasantly surprised to find that about a hundred of them wanted to do the cleanse! In order to stay accountable to each other, we created a Facebook group to keep one another motivated. So many people joined us simply because of the phenomenal results. In less than two months, about ten thousand people had joined the Facebook group and committed to doing the cleanse. In just ten short days, each of the participants and I lost ten to fifteen pounds, renewed our energy, reversed health conditions, and felt better than we had in years. Today the Facebook group has more than seven hundred thousand people supporting one another along their weight-loss journey. It has become more than just a support group for the Green Smoothie Cleanse—it's a supportive community for all those looking to lose weight and get healthy.

When I completed my first cleanse, I had lost eleven pounds. My energy was high, my skin was radiant, and my digestion and bloating had improved. I felt renewed and motivated again! Before I began the cleanse, I had been taking twenty-four supplements a day to help my body recover from mercury poisoning. Since completing the cleanse, I take only four supplements per day and have the greatest health and energy to achieve my life's dreams and goals. I learned that green smoothies are a great way to give the body the proper nutrition, not only to keep it healthy and vibrant but also to nourish the spark of life within it.

Fast-forward to today. Two million pounds have been lost on the Green Smoothie Cleanse, which I codified into a book, the #1 *New York Times* bestseller *10-Day Green Smoothie Cleanse.* The book's techniques are so successful and the word of mouth about the diet so organic, the book has been a perennial *New York Times* bestseller and we now have more than a million followers.

While the 10-Day Green Smoothie Cleanse is a great way to detox and jump-start weight loss, the 7-Day Apple Cider Vinegar Cleanse provides an alternative for even faster weight loss, particularly for those who don't want to drink green smoothies. The 7-Day Apple Cider Vinegar Cleanse is a different approach to weight loss that can be accomplished in a shorter period. So far, eighteen million people have followed my advice on using ACV to quickly lose weight and get healthy. For those who have less time, you can get the same results as on the other cleanse of losing up to fifteen pounds, but in just seven days. There are also some who simply do not love green smoothies, in taste or texture, but want to detox/cleanse; the ACV Cleanse is a great way to do so. To maximize your results, you can do both the ACV and Green Smoothie cleanses in a single month, and get an amazing jump-start to weight loss and greater health.

The ACV Cleanse will not only allow you to lose up to fifteen pounds in just one week, but will also reverse health conditions that plague you. The ACV Cleanse goes beyond weight loss and helps lower blood pressure, cholesterol, and blood sugar levels. By decreasing blood sugar, ACV lowers insulin levels, which leads to decreased fat in the body. Consuming apple cider vinegar will also improve gut health and enhance your skin. In fact, chapter 9 includes many additional uses for overall hair and skin health.

Congratulations on taking control of your health by caring for your body and feeding it what it needs to be slim, radiant, and energetic! If you're like me, you want to look and feel great, but it's not easy. Though we are surrounded by so many unhealthy yet enticing and addictive food choices, with the proper guidance and motivation, you can leave old eating patterns behind and establish new, healthier habits. I know how much courage it takes to begin a new life and relationship with food. I support you and encourage you in your efforts.

I suggest you read this book first for understanding, and then reread it with a mind to taking action and beginning your journey. Get a copy for a family member or friend so that you can encourage and support one another through this life-changing transformation. Your family, friends, and I will be here to guide you along and support you, which will be very helpful to you on this journey. Join seven hundred thousand others who access free support from me and my team on a daily basis on our Facebook page at https://www.facebook.com/groups/Green.Smoothie.Cleanse. That Facebook group is not just a support group about the green smoothie cleanse; it has become a support group for all those looking to lose weight and get healthy. You are not alone. We will do this together. Let your journey begin today.

Will you join me as we work together to heal the body, lose weight, and boost energy levels? By doing this, you will never have to worry about weight again. This is an amazing way to transform your body in just seven days. Get ready to start your 7-Day Apple Cider Vinegar Cleanse today!

chapter 1

What Is the 7-Day Apple Cider Vinegar Cleanse?

A cleanse is a short-term diet that detoxifies the body, increases energy, and jump-starts weight loss. The Apple Cider Vinegar Cleanse accomplishes all three of these in just one week. The 7-Day ACV Cleanse involves consuming apple cider vinegar for six days, along with "fasting with food," and using the seventh day as a transition day to break the cleanse. Instead of abstaining from food completely, such as in a traditional fast or water fast, you eat small amounts of food in a way that produces the therapeutic benefits of fasting—increased fat burning, lower blood sugar levels, and reduced inflammation—without the hunger. The 7-Day ACV Cleanse menu is low in carbs and protein but higher in fat. Your body stays nourished while also gaining the benefits of fasting. Long-term fasting can be harmful, but this seven-day cleanse is safe and effective.

The 7-Day Apple Cider Vinegar Cleanse will:

- Promote fat loss, both total body fat and body mass index (BMI)
- Improve digestion and overall gut health
- Decrease visceral fat—the fat around the waist and vital organs
- Help reverse diabetes as well as lower the risk of diabetes and insulin resistance by decreasing blood sugar levels
- Reduce inflammation by decreasing several inflammatory markers
- Decrease blood pressure and improve the health of your heart
- Lower cholesterol as you consume more foods high in heart-healthy fats
- Improve immune system function, a benefit of fasting for as little as four days

By combining "fasting with food" and ACV consumption, you will melt away body fat in the shortest possible time. We will take a closer look at both apple cider vinegar and fasting with food below.

APPLE CIDER VINEGAR

Apple cider vinegar comes from apples that have been crushed, distilled, and then fermented. The second stage of fermentation involves adding bacteria to convert the alcohol into vinegar. When the vinegar is mature, it will contain a cloudy substance called the "mother." The mother consists of dozens of strains of good bacteria. It also contains enzymes, which are essential for breaking down foods so that your body can use their nutrients. The concentrated bacteria and enzymes from the mother give ACV its antifungal, antiviral, and antibacterial properties, which help in healing the body.

Acetic acid makes up about 5 to 6 percent of apple cider vinegar. Although this is considered a relatively weak acid, it does have fairly strong acidic properties when concentrated. Apple cider vinegar also contains trace amounts of other acids, fiber, vitamins, and minerals.

Apple cider vinegar has been used for thousands of years for everything from soothing a sore throat to burning fat and improving blood sugar levels. Supported by scientific research, modern studies show that there are, indeed, numerous health benefits of apple cider vinegar.

The History of Apple Cider Vinegar

As noted above, the benefits of apple cider vinegar have been recognized for millennia. In both the American Civil War and World War I, apple cider vinegar was used to treat the wounds of soldiers on the battlefield. It has also been reported that Japanese samurai would drink it for strength, vitality, and power. Sometimes it's even used as a household cleaning product—where it's valued for its antibacterial qualities.

Modern science has provided plenty of evidence of apple cider vinegar's health benefits. In 2012, a Dutch study found that women in one North African culture who consumed a cup of apple cider vinegar daily achieved greater weight loss than women of that culture who did not.

The *Bioscience, Biotechnology, and Biochemistry* journal cited a Japanese study from 2014 that found the acetic acid in apple cider vinegar reduces body weight, body fat mass, and serum triglyceride levels, thereby reducing the risk for atherosclerosis in obese individuals. According to this study, adding one to two tablespoons of apple cider vinegar to your daily diet can help you lose more weight. The study also showed that drinking apple cider vinegar can reduce your body fat percentage, namely belly fat, in addition to lowering triglycerides.

A 2015 study demonstrated that apple cider vinegar consumption in patients with type 2 diabetes improved blood sugar control, and reduced insulin levels and high triglyceride levels. The acetic acid in ACV may promote fat burning, decrease blood sugar, and improve cholesterol levels.

How Apple Cider Vinegar Helps with Weight Loss

Acetic acid is apple cider vinegar's main active component. Multiple studies show that it has a favorable impact on weight loss in the following ways:

- *Lowers blood sugar.* A study by Carol Johnston, PhD, at Arizona State University showed that "drinking vinegar before eating actually led to a decrease in change of blood glucose post meals." This means that drinking apple cider vinegar before a high-carb meal can reduce blood sugar levels that typically occur after eating.

- *Helps you feel full longer.* A Swedish study found that when participants consumed apple cider vinegar with a meal, they reported feeling a higher level of satiety after eating than those who did not consume the vinegar. A higher level of satiety will prevent overeating and late-night snacking.

- *Reduces body fat.* A Japanese study was done showing that continuous apple cider vinegar intake reduces body weight, BMI, and body fat mass. This provides evidence of its ability to help prevent fat storage in the body.

- *Decreases insulin levels.* A study in the American Diabetes Association journal showed that consuming apple cider vinegar with a high-carb meal may improve insulin sensitivity after the meal, which helps to reduce fat storage in the body. This is especially beneficial to those who are insulin-resistant or those who have type 2 diabetes.

- *Improves metabolism.* A study done on rats showed that acetic acid caused an increase in the enzyme AMPK, which boosts one's metabolism by decreasing fat and sugar production in the liver.

- *Diminishes appetite.* Research done in the UK showed that acetic acid is a natural appetite suppressant because it

keeps our blood sugar levels steady, which minimizes cravings for sugar, carbs, and sweets.

While apple cider vinegar has a positive impact on weight loss,
the aforementioned studies show that it is most effective when
combined with other fasting methods, as discussed later in this
chapter.

Selecting an Apple Cider Vinegar

You want to buy organic, raw, unfiltered apple cider vinegar contain-
ing the mother (its presence should be indicated on the label). The
mother gives the vinegar a cloudy look, but do not be alarmed—this
ensures that the nutritional benefits are intact.

One popular brand is Bragg Organic Apple Cider Vinegar, but
my personal preference is White House.

How to Use Apple Cider Vinegar

Research shows that drinking one or two tablespoons of ACV in a
glass of water at bedtime or before meals aids in weight loss. When
acetic acid is in the gut, fat remains in the gut for a shorter period
of time. The acid also blocks enzymes that break down starchy
foods, which keep the fats and starches from being absorbed into
the body.

Ideally, dieters focused on losing weight, especially belly fat,
should ingest about three tablespoons of ACV per day in total—a

tablespoon before each meal, or two tablespoons in the morning and a tablespoon at bedtime. Taking it at bedtime will help lower blood sugar by morning, which leads to reduced fat storage in the body.

Important Warnings about Apple Cider Vinegar

1. Always dilute apple cider vinegar before consuming it, as it is highly acidic. If it is not diluted, it can burn the tissues in your mouth and throat, damaging your tooth enamel and stomach lining.

2. If ingesting apple cider vinegar causes you any stomach discomfort, discontinue its use.

3. Always rinse your mouth with water after ingesting apple cider vinegar to avoid damage to the tooth enamel.

4. If you are pregnant or nursing, consult your doctor and do your own research to determine if ACV is right for you.

5. Prior to using ACV on the skin, test a small patch of skin to detect any potential irritation or allergic reactions.

6. If you use prescription medications, consult your doctor to determine whether ACV is right for you or will interfere with your medication.

FASTING WITH FOOD

One of the most powerful tools on the planet for reducing body fat and reversing insulin resistance as well as many other health conditions is fasting. Fasting changes the way our hormones work by triggering our fat-burning hormones so that weight loss is easier. Simply put, the single greatest dietary intervention to reduce body fat and prevent disease is fasting.

Resetting your body to burn fat instead of being dependent on carbs and sugar can lead to weight loss and reverse all the symptoms associated with insulin resistance. It will also stabilize your blood sugar, lower blood pressure, boost your energy, and put you back in control of your appetite.

Our bodies are natural fat-burning machines. Due to our consumption of processed high-sugar foods, however, we have become dependent on carbs and sugar to supply us with energy. To lose weight, you need to reset your hormones and create the right environment for your body to burn stored energy—what we call body fat—in a process known as ketosis. Ketosis is when the body starts converting stored fat into ketones to use as fuel for the cells. Ketones are by-products of the body breaking down fat for energy.

Unfortunately, eating a lot of sugar and carbs means your body will never go into ketosis. Instead, your body will use the glucose from the carbohydrates as fuel instead of your stored body fat, so you remain overweight. However, by fasting you can "reset" your body to use stored body fat for fuel and lose the weight you desire. Once you begin fasting, your body will first burn through your glucose stores very quickly. Then, in less than twenty-four hours, your body will begin using stored body fat for fuel.

Many people think that you lose muscle when you fast. This is not true for short-term fasting of four to six days. In fact, studies show a slight increase in muscle mass after a typical five-day fast. This is because of an increase in growth hormones. Growth hormones are secreted by the pituitary gland at the base of your brain and play a key role in cellular repair and fat metabolism. You will not burn protein from muscle tissue while you fast until your body has run out of stored body fat.

Why Does Fasting Work?

Cutting carbs is one way to transition the body into ketosis; another way is through fasting. There are various forms of fasting, and there is a right way and a wrong way to fast to move the body into a state of ketosis. In fact, complete fasting with no food is unnecessary and can even be dangerous for people with diabetes, chronic kidney disease, and other health conditions.

The goal of fasting for dieters is to reduce calorie intake. However, fasting provides a range of benefits, such as weight loss, greater longevity, and improved health. Fasting is more effective than long-term, low-calorie dieting. Short-term, periodic fasting leads to increased weight loss, is easier to follow, and spares you the loss of muscle mass.

When you fast, blood glucose and insulin levels fall, which triggers the release of fat-burning hormones such as glucagon and adrenaline. These hormones cause the breakdown of fats called triglycerides that are stored in your fat tissue. Then, when triglycerides reach your liver, they are used to make ketones. When ketone levels rise to seven to eight millimoles per liter, you are officially in ketosis and your body starts converting stored fat into ketones to use as fuel for your cells. To confirm that your body is in ketosis, you can use keto sticks, also known as keto strips, which detect ketones in the urine. They are inexpensive, easy to use, and sold in most pharmacies. You get your results within one minute.

Cutting calories and working out are not the most expedient ways to lose weight. By fasting or reducing carbs, you can achieve ketosis, which tricks your metabolism into burning more fat.

The Benefits of Fasting

When you fast with food, you:

- Promote fat metabolism (weight loss) as well as *autophagy*, which is the body's way of cleaning out damaged cells in order to generate newer, healthier cells. Autophagy slows the aging process. You might hear autophagy referred to as "self-eating."

- Help lower blood pressure and cholesterol levels, stabilize blood sugar, improve gut health, and enhance skin health.

- Receive all the health benefits of fasting without the hunger because you are fasting with controlled types and amounts of food, which allows you to nourish your body while keeping it in a fasting state.

What You Can Expect

On the 7-Day Apple Cider Vinegar Cleanse, you will lose weight, preserve muscle, and reset your body's fat-burning hormones so the body can heal itself.

The positives:

- Fat loss, without any loss of muscle mass
- A significant reduction of abdominal fat
- Lower risk factors for various illnesses
- The ability to resist cravings for sweets, sugar, and carbs
- Glowing, younger-looking skin that is softer and healthier
- Increased energy and better mental clarity (sharpness of mind)
- Better quality of sleep

The negatives:

- Some people feel weak during the first two to three days of fasting.
- Most people feel hungry during the first few days due to reduced calories consumed.
- Some people get light headaches that will diminish after the first three days.

- There may be other detox symptoms, which we'll discuss in chapter 3.

After the 7-Day ACV Cleanse, we'll introduce *intermittent fasting,* a popular fasting method of not eating for a period of time, followed by eating within specified feeding windows. Intermittent fasting works by developing an eating pattern in which you alternate between periods of eating and fasting. Intermittent fasting is not about counting calories but rather about timing your meals. It does not say anything about which foods to eat but rather prescribes when you should eat them. The point of intermittent fasting is to prevent the body from producing insulin—therefore, no food should be consumed during the fasting time.

See chapter 4 for more details on intermittent fasting.

chapter 2

How to Do the 7-Day Apple Cider Vinegar Cleanse

The 7-Day Apple Cider Vinegar Cleanse involves fasting with food while drinking apple cider vinegar for six days, with the seventh day used as a transition day to break the fast. For the first six days, you will drink apple cider vinegar while also restricting calories. However, instead of abstaining from food completely, as you would with a traditional fast, you will eat small amounts of food in a way that produces the therapeutic benefits of fasting without the hunger. In short, you will be temporarily reducing the amount of food you typically eat for six days to take advantage of health benefits such as increased fat burning and reduced inflammation.

The ACV Cleanse follows a healthy regimen that is low in carbs and protein, while higher in fat. Your body will stay nourished with nutrients, while also gaining the health benefits of fasting. Remember, long-term fasting can be harmful, but this 7-Day ACV Cleanse is safer and more effective.

Preparing for the 7-Day Apple Cider Vinegar Cleanse

The 7-Day Apple Cider Vinegar Cleanse might be one of the greatest challenges of your life, but it is so worth it. This cleanse will challenge you spiritually, mentally, and physically. You will learn how to be more disciplined with your eating habits and improve your overall relationship with food.

The 7-Day Apple Cider Vinegar Cleanse will transform your health and help you shed pounds fast. Of course, there will be times when you feel frustrated or want to give up, but if you stick with it, your body will reward you for your efforts. You will be proud of yourself and delighted with your results at the end of the seven days.

Before you begin, it is important to mentally prepare for this journey. Each day, remember why you started and what your overall goals are: to get healthy and to lose weight. You can do this! You can take control of your health and weight and experience the joy of having your dream body.

Specific Guidelines for the ACV Cleanse

- One week before you begin, fortify your body with additional protein by ingesting protein shakes, powders, and drinks. Adding two scoops of your favorite protein powder per day should be sufficient.

- Purchase the key supplements (provided later in this chapter) required for the 7-Day ACV Cleanse. These supplements are critical to success and feeling comfortable during the cleanse.

- The daily calories for the first six days can be divided among breakfast, lunch, and dinner, or they can be taken as two meals and a snack. The ACV Cleanse is very flexible.

- Keep all eating within a twelve-hour period—for example, between 7 a.m. and 7 p.m., or between 9 a.m. and 9 p.m. Allow yourself two to three hours of NO EATING before bedtime—so if you go to sleep at 10 p.m., you'll want to stop eating by 7 or 8 p.m.

- Unlike most cleanses, you can have one cup of coffee or caffeinated green tea a day if necessary, though caffeine-free herbal teas are ideal.

- For the entire seven days, I recommend no intense workouts, long hot showers, or lengthy sun exposure. This is simply to avoid putting additional stress or strain on the body during times of intense cleansing or fasting.

Take Your Measurements and Photos

On the first day, weigh yourself and take your bust, waist, and hip measurements. Record these numbers along with the date. Some people will lose more weight while others will lose more inches, so you want to measure both! The majority of you will lose between five and fifteen pounds in seven days on the ACV Cleanse.

Next, take photos of your entire body and your face, close-up. This will enable you to document the physical changes that take place. Many times you will see a big difference in the whites of your eyes, along with reduced puffiness and dark circles. You will be able to monitor your progress not just by the weight on the scale but by how you look and feel overall. Off-the-scale victories allow you to celebrate changes that show your progress toward overall health goals so that the number on the scale is not your only way to track success.

Remember, this cleanse isn't just about weight loss, it's also about getting healthy. It is important to monitor your energy, digestion, moods, mental clarity, and skin. Let's get both the health and the weight-loss benefits of the ACV Cleanse! Don't let the scale demotivate you and become your enemy. Weight loss can fluctuate during a cleanse. In the end, you'll have lost weight.

Basic Eating Guidelines

Though I provide very specific food and menu options for each day of the Apple Cider Vinegar Cleanse later in this chapter, here are the basic eating guidelines that you will be following for the next seven days. They are pretty simple. On this program, you will eat foods that are low in protein, moderate in carbohydrates, and moderate in fats, but no animal products.

- Approximately 50 percent of your calories will come from healthy fats, such as olive oil, almonds, macadamia nuts, and other nuts and seeds.

- Approximately 45 percent of your calories will come from complex carbohydrate plant sources, including tomatoes, broccoli, sweet potatoes, and other choices listed in the menus below.

- Approximately 5 percent of your calories will come from plant-based protein sources.

- You will reduce the amount of sugar in your diet each day.

- You will ingest apple cider vinegar daily before meals or at bedtime.

Breakdown of Daily Calories

Day 1	Day 2	Day 3	Day 4	Day 5	Day 6	Day 7
1,200 Calories	1,200 Calories	800 Calories	800 Calories	800 Calories	800 Calories	Transition Day

Are You Over 250 Pounds?

If you weigh more than 250 pounds, it is okay to increase your calorie intake up to 1,400 calories on Days 1 and 2 and 1,000 calories on Days 3 through 6. If you need more calories, be sure you get what you feel your body needs. However, the typical calorie intake listed above is simple and easy to follow for most.

Days 1 and 2: 1,200 calories

- 600 calories from healthy fats (nuts, olive oil)
- 575 calories from complex carbohydrates (vegetables such as broccoli, tomatoes, sweet potatoes, etc.)
- 25 calories of plant-based protein

Days 3 to 6: 800 calories

- 400 calories from healthy fats (nuts, olive oil)
- 375 calories from complex carbohydrates (vegetables such as broccoli, tomatoes, sweet potatoes, etc.)
- 25 calories of plant-based protein

Day 7: Break the cleanse

The Menu

The good news is that you have options to choose from for all seven days of the cleanse.

1A: Days 1 and 2, Meal Plan A

- 1 cup quick oats, ample water, pinch of salt (all for oatmeal), 2 teaspoons butter (300 calories)
- 6 ounces carrots (about 18 baby carrots) (70 calories)
- Spinach Almond Salad: 2 cups spinach, ½ ounce roasted slivered almonds, 2 tablespoons light balsamic vinaigrette (145 calories). Note: You'll duplicate this salad later in the day.
- 2 ounces (about 24) macadamia nuts (404 calories)
- Spinach Almond Salad: 2 cups of spinach, ½ ounce roasted almonds/slivered, 2 tablespoons light balsamic vinaigrette (145 calories)
- 1½ ounces (about 50) dry-roasted peanuts (242 calories)
- 1 cup V8 vegetable juice (50 calories)
- JJ's Original ACV Detox Drink (10 calories)

Total: 1,366 calories

1B: Days 1 and 2, Meal Plan B

- 2 scrambled or fried eggs, 1 tablespoon extra-virgin olive oil, pinch of salt (270 calories)
- ¼ cup mashed avocado (100 calories)

- Spinach Strawberry Salad: 2 cups spinach, ½ ounce chopped pecans, ¼ cup sliced strawberries, 2 tablespoons light balsamic vinaigrette (185 calories). Note: You'll duplicate this salad later in the day.
- 1 cup V8 vegetable juice (50 calories)
- Spinach Strawberry Salad: 2 cups spinach, ½ ounce chopped pecans, ¼ cup sliced strawberries, 2 tablespoons light balsamic vinaigrette (185 calories)
- 2 ounces (about 24) macadamia nuts (404 calories)
- JJ's Original ACV Detox Drink (10 calories)

Total: 1,204 calories

2A: Days 3 to 6, Meal Plan A

- 2 scrambled or fried eggs, 1 tablespoon extra-virgin olive oil, pinch of salt (270 calories)
- ½ cup whole strawberries plus ½ cup blueberries (85 calories)
- 1 cup unsweetened almond milk (30 calories)
- ¼ cup mashed avocado (100 calories)
- 1 cup V8 vegetable juice (50 calories)
- 1 cup diced, steamed broccoli (50 calories)
- Spinach Almond Salad: 2 cups spinach, ½ ounce roasted slivered almonds, 2 tablespoons light balsamic vinaigrette (145 calories)
- ⅔ cup blueberries (80 calories)
- JJ's Original ACV Detox Drink (10 calories)

Total: 820 calories

2B: Days 3 to 6, Meal Plan B

- ½ cup dry quick oats, ample water, pinch of salt (all for oatmeal) (150 calories)
- 1 cup V8 vegetable juice (50 calories)
- 1 ounce (about 23) dry-roasted almonds (170 calories)
- ½ banana (50 calories)
- 10 dry-roasted macadamia nuts (180 calories)
- Spinach Almond Salad: 2 cups spinach, ½ ounce roasted slivered almonds, 2 tablespoons light balsamic vinaigrette (145 calories)
- ½ cup blueberries (60 calories)
- JJ's Original ACV Detox Drink (10 calories)

Total: 815 calories

2C: Days 3 to 6, Meal Plan C

- 1 cup quick oats, ample water, pinch of salt (all for oatmeal), 2 teaspoons butter (300 calories)
- 7 ounces (about 1 cup) canned spinach (60 calories)
- 1 cup whole strawberries (50 calories)
- 1½ ounces (about 50) dry-roasted peanuts (242 calories)
- 1 medium baked sweet potato, 1 teaspoon butter (135 calories)
- ¼ cup mashed avocado (100 calories)
- 1 cup V8 vegetable juice (50 calories)

- ¼ cup blueberries (30 calories)
- JJ's Original ACV Detox Drink (10 calories)

Total: 977 calories

Day 7: Transition Day

On the final day, you will transition into "soft" meals such as soup, veggies, salads, or green smoothies. Be sure to have complex carbohydrates (vegetables, fruits, etc.) and minimize the consumption of fish, meat, saturated fats, pastries, cheeses, milk, etc., for the day. The general thought is to eat clean and healthy, avoiding animal products and processed foods while focusing on the healthy options mentioned above. If you're a fan of green smoothies, this is a great day to have one.

Chapter 4 gives you guidelines on how to continue your success after Day 7.

It's important not to binge on food on Day 7. Gradually return to your normal foods over the next twelve hours. The pancreas and liver need to shift back into normal function after six days of fasting.

A popular transition meal you can have throughout the last day is Fat Burner Soup. This soup is packed with nutritional powerhouses such as sweet potatoes, spinach, garlic, carrots, and tomatoes. It flushes the fat away by restoring acid–alkaline and sodium–potassium balance to the body's organs and glands. The superfoods in this soup contain antioxidants and fiber, which aid in flushing toxins and, subsequently, fat from the body. The soup is warming and deliciously comforting.

Fat Burner Soup

1 medium sweet potato, peeled and cut into small
  cubes

3 carrots, peeled and sliced

1 celery rib, diced

1 small yellow onion, diced

1 teaspoon minced garlic (1 clove)

¼ teaspoon sea salt, or to taste

½ teaspoon black pepper

⅛ teaspoon allspice

1 teaspoon paprika

2 bay leaves

2 (15-ounce) cans kidney or navy beans, rinsed and
  drained

4 cups low-sodium vegetable broth

1 (14.5-ounce) can diced tomatoes (no salt added)

4 cups baby spinach, loosely packed

1 tablespoon extra-virgin olive oil, for serving only
  (optional)

1. Place the sweet potato, carrots, celery, onion, garlic, salt, pepper, allspice, paprika, bay leaves, beans, broth, and tomatoes in a slow cooker or large pot. Cover and cook on low heat for 6 to 8 hours.
2. Add the spinach, and continue cooking for 5 to 7 minutes, or until the spinach is wilted.
3. Ladle the soup into bowls and drizzle with a little olive oil, if desired, to enhance the flavor and help the body absorb the nutrients.

To make a thicker soup, you can mash some of the vegetables with a fork once they are tender (typically after 5 to 7 hours). Another option is to remove 1 to 1½ cups of the soup (liquid only). However, most enjoy it as is.

After the 7-Day ACV Cleanse, I will introduce *intermittent fasting*, an eating pattern where you alternate between periods of eating and fasting. See chapter 4 for details.

What to Drink on the 7-Day Apple Cider Vinegar Cleanse

The ACV Cleanse has a lot of flexibility. The following drinks are recommended:

- Daily ACV Detox Drink (see details below for the most important drink on the cleanse)
- Plenty of water (not fruit-infused water)
- Decaffeinated herbal teas
- One cup of coffee or green tea per day with a splash of nondairy creamer and stevia

What Is Not Allowed

- Alcohol
- Sodas, including diet sodas
- Juices
- Coconut water
- Cow's milk

Daily ACV Detox Drink

There are two recipes for the Daily ACV Detox Drink.

JJ's Original ACV Detox Drink

This drink gets rid of bloating, indigestion, and belly fat!

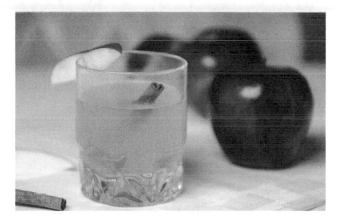

2 tablespoons apple cider vinegar

Dash of cayenne pepper

Squeeze of lemon juice

1 packet stevia (optional)

1. Fill a mason jar or glass with 8 to 12 ounces of water.
2. Add the vinegar, cayenne, lemon juice, stevia (if using).
3. Stir and enjoy, and keep the unused portion refrigerated.

You can add stevia to taste. Avoid honey, as that adds natural sugar, which can work against weight loss.

JJ's Berry Apple Cider Vinegar Drink

If you don't love the taste of JJ's Original ACV Detox Drink, try this variation.

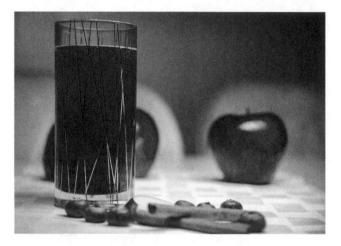

2 tablespoons apple cider vinegar

2 tablespoons mixed berries, mashed

1 tablespoon lemon juice

1 packet stevia

1. Fill a mason jar or glass with 20 to 24 ounces of water.
2. Add the vinegar, berries, lemon juice, and stevia.
3. Stir and enjoy. Refrigerate the unused portion.

Sample 7-Day Regimen for the Apple Cider Vinegar Cleanse

Day	Meal Plan	Drinks	Supplements
Day 1	1B	ACV Drink, Coffee, Herbal Tea, Water	Electrolytes, Omega-3, Vitamin B Complex
Day 2	1B	ACV Drink, Coffee, Herbal Tea, Water	Electrolytes, Omega-3, Vitamin B Complex
Day 3	2A	ACV Drink, Coffee, Herbal Tea, Water	Electrolytes, Omega-3, Vitamin B Complex
Day 4	2B	ACV Drink, Coffee, Herbal Tea, Water	Electrolytes, Omega-3, Vitamin B Complex
Day 5	2A	ACV Drink, Coffee, Herbal Tea, Water	Electrolytes, Omega-3, Vitamin B Complex
Day 6	2B	ACV Drink, Coffee, Herbal Tea, Water	Electrolytes, Omega-3, Vitamin B Complex
Day 7	Fat Burner Soup	ACV Drink, Coffee, Herbal Tea, Water	Electrolytes, Omega-3, Vitamin B Complex

Complete Your 7-Day ACV Cleanse Regimen

Day	Meal Plan	Drinks	Supplements
Day 1			
Day 2			
Day 3			
Day 4			
Day 5			
Day 6			
Day 7			

Who Should Not Do the 7-Day ACV Cleanse?

There are certain individuals for whom this cleanse is not ideal:

- Pregnant women
- People over the age of seventy, unless in extremely good health

- People who are suffering from any disease of the liver or kidney
- Underweight people and anyone suffering from anorexia with an extremely low body mass index (BMI)
- Athletes during competition or intense training sessions

An Important Warning

People who MUST get their doctor's approval before they start:

- Anyone who takes insulin or medications that lower blood sugar levels
- Anyone with hypertension, cancer, or a cardiovascular, neurodegenerative, or autoimmune disease

How Often Can You Do the 7-Day ACV Cleanse?

- If you are overweight or obese, it's fine to do the cleanse once a month.

- If you are at a normal weight but struggle with various health conditions, then every other month is ideal.

- If you are healthy with no significant concerns, and at your ideal weight, then once every three months is recommended.

Supportive Supplements

Listed below are the supplements that are highly recommended. These supplements will ensure that you do not suffer from any nutritional deficiencies and will minimize detox symptoms.

- A mineral/electrolyte supplement will ensure that specific bodily functions run at optimal levels. My favorite brands are Dr. Berg's Electrolyte Powder and Ultima Replenisher.

- An omega-3 supplement increases heart-healthy fats during the cleanse. My favorite brands are Nature Made and NOW.

- A vitamin B complex will help you maintain healthy energy levels throughout the day. My favorite brands are Divine Bounty and Nature Made.

- Powdered green drinks, such as Green Vibrance, are a superfood supplement that provide additional micronutrients (optional).

Shopping List for the 7-Day ACV Cleanse

- Quick oats/unsweetened oatmeal
- Eggs (1 dozen)
- Spinach, fresh (large container)
- Carrots
- Broccoli
- Sweet potato

- Avocados (2)
- Strawberries (1 pint)
- Blueberries (1 pint)
- Bananas
- Almonds (slivered), macadamia nuts, dry-roasted peanuts, pecans (chopped)
- Canned spinach (about 8 ounces)
- Extra-virgin olive oil (small bottle)
- V8 vegetable juice (large bottle)
- Light balsamic vinaigrette (e.g., Newman's Own)
- Apple cider vinegar

Optional

- Unsweetened almond milk
- Stevia
- Lemon juice
- Cayenne pepper

Optional, but highly recommended

- Supportive supplements (electrolytes, omega-3, and vitamin B complex)

chapter 3

JJ's Personal Tips for Success

Here are a few tips that will help you maximize your results on the 7-Day Apple Cider Vinegar Cleanse.

Preparation is key to success. It's important to spend the first week preparing for success. This includes reading the book for understanding, completing your grocery shopping for foods and supplements, and beginning the supplement regimen one week prior to starting the cleanse. These activities will make the cleanse easier and ensure you get the best results.

Don't get wrapped around the axle. The 7-Day Apple Cider Vinegar Cleanse is a very flexible plan. There are different menu options for each day. You can eat everything as three meals or as two meals plus snacks, whichever works best for your schedule. You don't need to fixate on the exact number of carbs, proteins, and fats since the daily menus have already been calculated at the macronutrient level to ensure the best results. The most important factor is to keep all eating within a twelve-hour period—for example, between 7 a.m. and 7 p.m., or between 9 a.m. and 9 p.m. Remember to avoid late-night eating. Allow yourself two to three hours of NO EATING before bedtime.

Take it easy and get plenty of rest. For the entire seven days, I recommend no intense workouts, long hot showers, or lengthy sun exposure. Athletes doing intense workouts or in competition should avoid the ACV Cleanse altogether. However, light exercise, such as walking or restorative yoga, is fine.

Increase your protein intake one week prior to starting. To ensure you maintain the right nutritional balance, you'll want to increase your protein intake before starting the ACV Cleanse. An easy way to add protein without the extra calories is with protein powder drinks. Adding two scoops of your favorite protein powder to water per day for seven days prior to the cleanse should be sufficient. My favorite brands are Ancient Nutrition Bone Broth Protein and Nutiva Hemp Protein as a vegan alternative.

Don't stalk the scale. On any cleanse or fast, you may gain on some days, while other days you may lose weight. This is perfectly normal. Weight fluctuates due to three things in the body: muscle, fat, and water. Muscle weighs the most—that's why you can work out and build muscle and thereby *gain* weight. You are actually making progress by building muscle, since it will help you burn fat all day long.

For women, water is the biggest culprit, due to our hormones. Many of us gain five to ten pounds of water weight during our cycle.

For some, excess salt/sodium causes water to be trapped under the tissue in the body, making us weigh more and appear bloated and puffy. Don't sweat it if your weight is a little up and down. (Only if it's up every week, week after week, do you have a problem.) Look into getting a Tanita scale—it will tell you not just your weight but also the percentage of muscle, fat, and water in your body, which is helpful for people who work out.

Drink plenty of water. At a minimum, drink sixty-four ounces of water per day, as it helps to flush out toxins. If you're drinking enough water, you will urinate frequently when you begin this cleanse, and that is a good thing. The general rule of thumb is to drink half your body weight in ounces. So, as an example, if you weigh 180 pounds, you would drink ninety ounces of water per day.

Drink herbal, decaffeinated teas. Herbal teas are an important addition to your cleanse. Not only will herbal teas help you feel less hungry, they can also aid the metabolic processes in the body. Good herbal teas to include are chamomile, peppermint, dandelion root, ginger, milk thistle, sarsaparilla, and ginseng.

Keep your bowels moving. As your body adjusts to the daily regimen of the 7-Day ACV Cleanse, your digestive system may need assistance and you may need help moving your bowels the first few days. Ideally, you should move your bowels one to three times per day and never less than once a day.

If you haven't had a bowel movement in more than twenty-four hours, there are two methods to get things moving.

Method 1: Use the saltwater flush, which involves drinking

uniodized sea salt with water. To tolerate the taste and make it go down, mix two teaspoons of sea salt into eight ounces of water; immediately after drinking this, follow with three more eight-ounce glasses of water. Do this first thing in the morning while you have an empty stomach, and you will have several bowel movements within thirty minutes to an hour.

Method 2: One product that works wonders at removing the old fecal matter in your colon is Mag 07, which I highly recommend. Take three to four pills at bedtime and you can look forward to a heavy bowel movement in the morning. Many of my clients use Mag 07 for regular colon cleansing.

Take the time to address emotional eating. During the 7-Day ACV Cleanse, the restrictive regimen will be challenging if you struggle with emotional eating. This is a great time to address this issue and improve your relationship with food. To deal with your emotions, you must come to understand that the bad experiences that happened in your life have probably been floating around in your mind for years. We often try to suppress these feelings; therefore, they have never been properly processed. It's time to stop using food to soothe, comfort, calm, and distract you from unpleasant emotions and feelings.

Sad or painful experiences teach us lessons we need to learn so that we can grow and mature—they are not meant to linger for years and years. Just as we can rid our bodies of toxic waste, we can rid it of toxic emotions. Instead of eating to distract ourselves from bad feelings, we need to process and eliminate them—just like the body does with food: it takes the nutrients it needs and expels the rest.

Consider seeing a therapist and reading my book *Think Yourself*

Thin: A 30-Day Guide to Permanent Weight Loss to deal with emotional eating and other struggles that have kept you from reaching your goal weight.

Get support from family and friends. Our eating habits are greatly influenced by our culture and by those closest to us. Think about the people you eat with most often: family, friends, and lovers. For many of us, food equals fun. We eat to socialize, celebrate, and show love to one another. How many people eat healthy right up until they are around their family and friends? Our loved ones have the strongest influence on how successful we will be in changing our habits and living a healthy lifestyle. They often encourage us to indulge or tell us we look good and don't need to be on a diet.

Whenever we tell someone we love that we are making changes to improve our health, their response will likely have a large effect on whether we succeed or fail. Studies show that people who do not have support from loved ones are less successful in achieving their life goals. When you communicate to a family member that you are trying to lose weight, it is essential that they show support and encouragement. They should understand that your new lifestyle is important to you. You will have a harder time succeeding if they do the opposite, or criticize your food choices. This disagreement will become a source of stress and tension in the relationship. The ideal situation is when a family member decides to change their behavior along with you. That way, you can hold each other accountable.

It is also very helpful to interact with others who are doing the same cleanse. You can meet such people and get encouragement and tips from me and thousands of others by joining my Facebook support group: https://www.facebook.com/groups/

Green.Smoothie.Cleanse. We start the 7-Day Apple Cider Vinegar Cleanse every other month.

Get comfortable with being uncomfortable. For the first two or three days, you will feel tired, hungry, and irritable. These feelings are normal and should be expected. Know that your body is receiving sufficient nutrients each day and look for alternative ways to feel satisfied beyond eating. You must focus on getting your body through this seven-day process in order to break unhealthy eating habits. Your body has the natural ability to maintain its ideal weight if you focus on healthy living. As the days go by, you will feel more energetic and desire less food. You will also learn to eat in moderation, as you train your body to have better eating habits. Go through the process, be uncomfortable from time to time, and let your body reward you for your efforts.

Follow the daily menus as provided. To make the 7-Day Apple Cider Vinegar Cleanse safe, easy, and most effective, adhere to the daily regimen provided, which offers more than one option to choose from each day. You may find that you enjoy eating certain foods you thought you didn't like at all. You will gain discipline, focus, and strength as each day passes. If you are allergic to one of the foods on the daily menu, replace it with more of the other foods on the daily meal plan. Be mindful of matching the calorie count so that you don't exceed your daily calorie limit.

Engage in positive self-talk. Thoughts and feelings turn into actions, and actions into reality. Remember, you are beginning a new chapter in your life. Let me encourage you right now to get started with your journey. Many ask, "How do I start?" or "How do I get there?" Well, it begins with positive self-talk. You must stop thinking and speaking negatively about yourself. You are not fat, lazy, ugly, or sick. Your true self is naturally thin, beautiful, and healthy. If you have negative thoughts about yourself, you'll attract negative people and outcomes into your life. If you say that you will never lose weight, you're exactly right: you won't. If you say you can, your subconscious mind believes and begins to move your actions in the direction of losing weight.

Focus on health, and you'll never have to worry about weight again. If you're doing the cleanse for fast weight loss, you're totally missing the additional benefits. Don't let the scale become your enemy! Most people lose between five and fifteen pounds on the ACV Cleanse; however, you'll want to focus on your overall health, and look at your digestion, skin/complexion, and mental clarity for improvements. The long-term focus is on healthy living. Target getting healthy, and the weight loss will follow.

Make your health a priority. You must begin to think differently. First, decide that your health is one of the top priorities in your life. Know that your body is naturally thin. If you prepare your mind and absorb the knowledge offered in this book, you will have the power you need to become your best self and transform your life in every way. Even if you are a busy mom or a high-powered career executive, know that today begins the journey toward your most amazing, healthy self. It is time to treat your body as the greatest gift that you have. It is time to shine as the person you were always meant to be. When you have a positive energy in life, love, joy, success, and wealth come your way. Every interaction at work, church, home, or in the street can be simply magnetic. Get healthy, lose weight, and watch your entire life begin to change for the better.

ACV Cleanse Detox Symptoms

Detox symptoms are a natural reaction that your body undergoes when switching from burning glucose (sugar) to burning fat instead (similar to withdrawal from drugs or alcohol). Typical symptoms include:

- Sugar cravings
- Dizziness/confusion
- Rash
- Brain fog/poor focus and concentration
- Irritability
- Stomach pain/nausea
- Cramping
- Muscle soreness
- Difficulty falling asleep

These symptoms are temporary and a normal reaction to entering ketosis. The detox symptoms should resolve after the completion of the cleanse.

To minimize detox symptoms, be sure to drink plenty of water to release toxins, use electrolytes to help the body stay hydrated, avoid intense exercise, and get more rest during the ACV Cleanse.

How to Continue Weight Loss after the 7-Day Apple Cider Vinegar Cleanse: Intermittent Fasting

You've just finished the 7-Day Apple Cider Vinegar Cleanse, you've lost up to fifteen pounds, and you feel great! You want to keep this going—so now what? Do the ACV Cleanse again? Of course, you could do another cleanse in a month, but you can't keep doing them back-to-back. The cleanse is a great way to jump-start your weight loss and transition away from sugary foods and carbohydrate-filled diets. However, its primary purpose is to detoxify and heal the body, and losing weight is just one of the many benefits.

This chapter will tell you exactly what to do after the 7-Day Apple Cider Vinegar Cleanse and why. After reading this chapter and putting it into action, you will have not only a powerful approach to eating but also a way to detox your body, improve your health, increase mental strength, and help naturally balance your hormones. Here you'll learn more about why each of the previously mentioned facets is important to your weight-loss journey. The bottom line is that you will be able to continue losing weight while moving toward achieving optimum health.

In this chapter, we will discuss:

- How intermittent fasting is defined
- The science of intermittent fasting
- Benefits of intermittent fasting
- Common myths about intermittent fasting
- How to do intermittent fasting

What Is Intermittent Fasting?

Intermittent fasting is when you eat during a specific period of time, and you fast the rest of the time. During the times you eat, you have very few restrictions as to what foods you can eat. However, the healthier you eat, the better the results will be. During the fasting window, you are not allowed to consume any food/calories. You should drink lots of water and enjoy black coffee and teas during the fasting window.

Intermittent fasting focuses more on the time during which you eat as opposed to the amount of calories you consume. It does not dictate which foods to eat but rather *when* you should eat them. The point of intermittent fasting is to prevent the body from producing insulin—therefore, no food should be consumed during the fasting time. It is not a diet but an eating pattern to reduce your blood sugar, turn on your fat-burning hormones, and use your stored fats as fuel so that you lose weight faster.

With intermittent fasting, you will first notice that you are hungrier. Once your body adjusts to fasting daily, your insulin levels will drop and your brain will stop sending signals that you need to eat. In other words, the longer you maintain a regular fasting method, the easier it becomes. With intermittent fasting, your mind-set about eating becomes more purposeful as you focus on your eating versus fasting windows. Intermittent fasting becomes so easy and natural to maintain that you begin wondering why you haven't eaten this way all along.

Keep in mind that *fasting* is a broad term—it can mean anything from not eating for days (water fast) to skipping one meal a day to only eating soup. As far as intermittent fasting goes, there are many different options with their own protocols and pros/cons. All the intermittent fasting methods lead to weight loss and improved health; however, the one I recommend for its effectiveness and ease of practice is the 16:8 method. This method's eating schedule consists of a sixteen-hour fast and an eight-hour feasting period. When I refer to intermittent fasting going forward, I always mean the 16:8 method.

Each day, you eat healthy during the eight-hour window and fast during the sixteen-hour window. But keep in mind that the majority of the sixteen-hour fast happens while you are sleeping. An example of a 16:8 fast would be that you eat no foods after 8 p.m., then skip breakfast and resume eating after noon the next day. Or else you might choose to eat between 10 a.m. and 6 p.m., which allows plenty of time for a healthy breakfast, lunch around midday, and a light dinner or snack around 5 or 5:30 p.m. before starting your fast. It's important to maintain a consistent schedule of fasting/eating times to avoid disrupting your hormones. So pick a schedule that's convenient for you and try to stick with it daily.

As with all eating or nutritional programs, check with your doctor for approval before beginning intermittent fasting. Although the 16:8 plan is very safe for healthy, well-nourished people, it doesn't suit the following individuals:

- People with a history of eating disorders
- People with type 1 diabetes
- Pregnant women or nursing mothers
- People who are malnourished or underweight
- Women with fertility issues

Intermittent Fasting and the DHEMM System

Years ago, I developed a comprehensive approach to not only weight loss but greater overall health and well-being. It is called the DHEMM System, which stands for Detox, Hormonal Balance, Eat Clean, Mental Mastery, and Move, as described below.

- DETOX: Use several (no fewer than three) of the twenty-one detox methods weekly (detailed in the *Green Smoothies for Life* book by JJ Smith).
- HORMONAL BALANCE: Optimize your hormones for weight loss.
- EAT CLEAN: Eat healthy, whole, and unprocessed foods.
- MENTAL MASTERY: Achieve the right mental focus to stay motivated.
- MOVE: Get moving and increase your physical activity.

Intermittent fasting is so powerful that it addresses four out of the five pillars of the DHEMM system, which are detoxing, balancing hormones, eating clean, and mental mastery. The DHEMM System and intermittent fasting are very complementary to each other.

The Science of Intermittent Fasting

Although fasting has been around since biblical times, we are just beginning to fully understand what happens to our bodies when we fast and how it affects our health. The first thing your body does when you are not eating is change your hormone levels so that the body can continue to receive fuel for energy. After about twelve hours of fasting (no eating at all), the glucose from the food you ate most recently is depleted. As your glucose levels continue to drop, your pancreas no longer needs to produce insulin to keep your blood sugar under control.

When your insulin levels are lower, your stored body fat becomes readily available to be used as fuel. Once your body can no longer find glucose, it resorts to the glycogen stores in your liver and muscles. After the glycogen is consumed, it then turns to stored body fat. Once this happens, the fatty acids produce ketones to provide energy for both your brain and your body.

As your insulin levels decrease, levels of human growth hormone (HGH) begin to increase. Growth hormones are secreted by the pituitary gland at the base of your brain and play a key role in cellular repair and fat metabolism. Some studies have shown that fasting for twelve hours increases your growth hormones by 30 percent, while fasting for sixteen hours gives a rise of 200 percent. Increasing your HGH helps to burn stored fat as well as prevent muscle loss.

In the fasting state, your cells will start repairing; this is known as autophagy. Autophagy is the body's way of cleaning out damaged cells in order to generate newer, healthier cells. During repair, autophagy detoxifies the body and slows down aging. The process can begin as early as twelve hours into a fast. This will target and eliminate cells that may be full of toxins, bacteria, viruses, and other debris. Fasting is a great way to detox the body and repair cellular damage.

Benefits of Intermittent Fasting

Intermittent fasting is both a weight-loss and a health phenomenon. You should expect to experience the following benefits:

Permanent Weight Loss

The most obvious reason for weight loss is that you will be eating fewer meals, resulting in fewer overall calories per day. Assuming that you do not overeat during the eating window, you will notice consistent weight loss. One reason it works for permanent weight loss is that the hormonal changes that occur during intermittent fasting improve your metabolic function, allowing your body to use more fat and stay in fat-burning mode. The great news is that you don't even need to count calories, since intermittent fasting isn't about what you eat as much as when you eat. In recent studies that compared obese individuals on an intermittent fasting plan with others on a traditional diet plan, both groups were able to achieve a lower body mass index (BMI), but the intermittent fasting group showed a greater tendency to keep the weight off after a year. This is ideal, as it breaks the cycle of "losing and gaining" with which many dieters struggle.

Improved Brain Function

When you skip breakfast and fast in the morning, you will experience increased mental clarity and begin to feel as if you have improved brain function. There's a reason for this. You may have heard the term *brain fog*, describing the inability to think clearly and concentrate. It happens most often in the mornings, particularly at the beginning of your workday. We often compensate by drinking more and more coffee. Blood sugar spikes are often the reason you experience brain fog. The solution is to skip breakfast and start your day with fasting. Studies show that the process of autophagy creates pathways to establish new neurons in the brain. Autophagy is complemented by brain-derived neurotropic factor (BDNF), a protein that impacts the function of the brain and the peripheral nervous system. Fasting increases BDNF, which then supports existing brain cells while also stimulating the growth of new neurons in the brain.

Enhanced Spiritual Life

Intermittent fasting involves an element of sacrifice. Giving up your morning routines and habits such as breakfast requires you to deny the flesh. With intermittent fasting, you begin to focus inwardly and pay less attention to what to eat when you awaken. Even as you experience hunger pangs, you will have to find a quiet place to reflect and take your mind off food and eating. You will also feel lighter physically and spiritually. You can use the fasting window for prayer and self-reflection to avoid the temptation of food. For many, intermittent fasting will feel as if you are making a sacrifice by suffering a little, which builds spiritual fortitude. Allow your body to become content without food, other temptations, and the burdens of this world.

Stimulation of Fat-Burning Hormones

Intermittent fasting causes a reboot of your fat-burning hormones. When you fast, your pancreas takes a break from producing insulin, while your pituitary gland sends out an additional supply of human growth hormone, a vital hormone for cell regeneration. Your body burns more fat and increases muscle mass when you produce higher levels of HGH. Additionally, the digestive organs are able to rest as you avoid eating and, thus, digesting foods. This is important because the digestive system plays such a key role in keeping your metabolism revved up.

Reduced Risk of Diabetes

As you become overweight or obese, you increase your risk of type 2 diabetes. There is a correlation between weight gain and insulin resistance, which leads to type 2 diabetes. When you become insulin-resistant, your pancreas does not produce enough insulin to keep your blood sugar under control. High blood sugar levels increase the risk of developing type 2 diabetes. Maybe this has already happened to you. The good news is that intermittent fasting will lower insulin resistance so that the blood sugar drops by 4 to 6 percent. More importantly, insulin levels also decrease by as much as 20 to 30 percent.

Common Myths about Intermittent Fasting

There are many misconceptions about intermittent fasting. Here are the most common myths:

Myth 1: You will lose muscle mass.

You may have heard that once you go into starvation mode, you'll lose muscle mass, but studies show that this is not true when intermittent fasting is done correctly. As mentioned, intermittent fasting causes an increase in growth hormones, which reduces the chance of losing muscle mass. In fact, your metabolic rate actually increases during short periods of fasting. Your body uses stored fats for fuel when you are not eating. Skipping a meal or two does not count as starvation. You would have to go for at least thirty-six hours without eating for your body to be in starvation mode. After that first thirty-six hours, it would take an additional twelve hours before your body began to experience any muscle loss. Even if you decided to go through long periods of fasting (for several days), you could eat a high-protein meal just before you began in order to supply your bloodstream with a sufficient amount of amino acids to prevent muscle degradation. Therefore you can dismiss the fear of losing muscle mass during intermittent fasting and focus on creating your best body.

Myth 2: You must eat five to six small meals a day to lose weight.

It's true that your body does need some energy to digest food, as you burn about 10 percent of your calories on digestion alone. However, studies show that how often one eats has no effect on overall calorie burn during the day. Therefore eating more meals throughout the day does not enhance calorie burn. Additionally, some believe that eating protein five to six times per day supports the development of muscles. However, studies show that the total amount of protein consumed in a day, not spacing out consumption every few hours, is what is necessary to build and maintain muscle mass. Frequent meals *will* allow you to avoid hunger pangs, but this can also be managed through self-control and discipline.

Myth 3: Intermittent fasting will cause you to gain weight.

The thought is that you will be so hungry from fasting that you will overeat during the eating window. However, this depends on the individual, and most people do not try to overcompensate for the meals missed while fasting. You definitely do not want to overindulge because you haven't eaten for a long period of time. Once your body adjusts to fasting on a daily basis, you will maintain a normal diet during your eight-hour eating window.

Myth 4: You are starving yourself.

You may have heard that intermittent fasting is starving yourself and harmful to your health. Some believe that you are depriving your body of vital nutrients that you need to stay healthy. Understand, there is a difference between "starving" and simply "being hungry." Starvation is when you do not have sufficient food for the body to function. It means you are restricting calories without a choice and there is no food in your future. With intermittent fasting, you are purposely choosing to avoid meals/calories for a specified period, but there is a plan to resume eating after that time. It would take several days of no eating at all to have your body go into starvation mode, which does slow down your metabolism. The 16:8 intermittent fasting method only restricts eating for sixteen hours per day, and this will not put you into starvation mode nor slow your metabolism.

How to Do Intermittent Fasting

Here is a quick summary of the guidelines that will ensure your success while doing intermittent fasting (16:8).

- Each day, you choose healthy options during the eight-hour eating window, then fast during the sixteen-hour window—much of which happens while you are asleep. You might decide to eat between 10 a.m. and 6 p.m., giving yourself plenty of time for a healthy breakfast, lunch, and then a light dinner or snack just before starting your fast.

Or perhaps you prefer to eat no foods after 8 p.m. and skip breakfast the next morning, then resume eating after noon. It's important to maintain a consistent schedule of fasting/ eating times to avoid disrupting your hormones. Pick a schedule and stick with it daily.

- To maximize results, during your eight-hour eating window, you should eat clean and healthy, focusing on high protein, low carbs, and moderate healthy fats. You could have pizza and burgers from time to time, but most of your calories should come from whole, healthy foods. *Keep in mind that we provide some healthy and flavorful recipes that you can eat during the 8-hour eating window in chapter 6.*

- While fasting, you should drink plenty of fluids. Pure water is ideal, but you can also have black coffee, green tea, herbal teas, and other no-calorie beverages. Water with lemon, apple cider vinegar, or stevia is fine, as well as any sugar-free carbonated waters. Staying hydrated will also keep the hunger pangs away.

- There is flexibility during your eating window. You could eat two meals or three, as long as you keep all eating within the eight-hour window.

- When it comes to working out, you may think that the sixteen-hour fasting window is not the ideal time for physical activity, especially if, like many people, you prefer food or a protein shake just prior to working out. However, if you are able to, you can work out a few hours before breaking your fast in order to trigger the release of more growth hormones while your insulin levels are low.

Intermittent fasting can help you live longer. Studies have shown that simply by restricting the number of calories you consume every day, you will lengthen your life span. Intermittent fasting is easy once you realize that you do not have to pay so much attention to food in order to lose weight. It is a routine that one can easily adopt and see great success.

5 Ways to Accelerate Weight Loss on the 7-Day Apple Cider Vinegar Cleanse

The 7-Day Apple Cider Vinegar Cleanse is about improving the quality of your life and health as you age. It helps you achieve three things:

- *Weight loss:* Losing fat fast, without losing muscle mass.
- *Vibrancy:* Staying vital and maintaining good health as you age.
- *Youthfulness:* Staying youthful well beyond what is typically expected.

If you follow the plan, you will achieve the benefits and set yourself on a path to healthy living. There are several actions you can take to accelerate your results on the ACV Cleanse. I often call these my five "weight-loss hacks" because they are little-known secrets to helping the body burn fat and lose weight faster.

Keep in mind that these methods are *optional* and are not required for success on the ACV Cleanse. However, they will enhance your results, so feel free to incorporate any or all of them into this program. You can add all of these hacks to your daily regimen to create an even healthier body as you get slimmer.

1. Alkaline water
2. Liver cleansing
3. Digestive cleansing
4. Coffee and green tea
5. Fiber

Alkaline Water

It is important to stay hydrated, especially when fasting and dieting. Dehydration can lead to unclear thinking, mood changes, bloating, and constipation. Water is involved in every type of cellular process in the body. If you are dehydrated, all of these processes run less efficiently, including your metabolism. By drinking enough water, you regulate how much you eat as well as aid the body in proper digestion. A study published in *Obesity* found that overweight adults who drank sixteen ounces of water thirty minutes before their meals lost nine more pounds at the end of a twelve-week period compared to those who didn't drink any water before meals. Ideally, you should drink half your body weight in ounces.

My favorite type of water to enhance hydration is alkaline water.

Alkaline water has a higher pII level (eight or nine) than regular drinking water (six or seven). The pH level measures how acidic or alkaline a substance is on a scale of zero to fourteen. For example, something with a pII of one would be very acidic, and something with a pH of thirteen or fourteen would be very alkaline. Your overall pH balance is extremely important to determining good health. The goal is a healthy state of alkalinity. Many experts say that disease cannot exist when the body is in an alkaline state. When the body is in an acidic state, it is not healthy. An acidic body puts you at greater risk for all kinds of disease, chronic illness, and weight gain. Drinking alkaline water (ion water or hydrogen-rich water) can help to keep the body in an alkaline state, detoxifies the body, increases energy levels, and leaves the skin looking smoother, more elastic, and more youthful.

A simple way to make your water more alkaline is to add a squeeze of lemon or lime to a glass of distilled water. It is important to use distilled water because tap water may have additives or artificial ingredients. You can also purchase pH drops and add them to your water to boost its pH level.

You can also purchase alkaline water in health food stores or buy a portable alkaline water bottle (such as an IonPod) that converts regular water to alkaline water. There are also machines that convert the water from your faucet to alkaline water, but these are much more expensive—a Kangen machine, for example, costs close to $5,000.

You should not drink alkaline water with meals, though any other time throughout the day is fine. You must gradually build up your body's tolerance to alkaline water, beginning with a small amount of about eight ounces a day. If you drink too much alkaline water too quickly, you will have strong detox symptoms, such as headaches or rashes. Work your way up slowly until you use alkaline water as your primary water to meet your daily water-intake goals.

Liver Cleansing

The key to losing weight and keeping it off is to keep the liver healthy and operating at peak performance. The liver is the number-one secret weapon in achieving weight loss. The liver is responsible for eliminating and neutralizing toxins in the body while also breaking down fats. Therefore it is essential that we cleanse the liver to improve the body's detoxification capabilities and to help the body metabolize and burn fats.

Although there are several organs of elimination in the body, most health practitioners agree that the liver is the primary one. It has been said that the length and quality of life depends on proper liver function. The liver works day and night to cleanse the blood of toxins such as unhealthy chemicals, bad bacteria, and other foreign substances. The liver is also responsible for metabolizing fats. As such, it is critical to keep the liver as clean as possible.

When your liver functions efficiently, it is much easier for you to lose weight. The liver has to perform well enough to eliminate the toxins that are causing fat cells in the body. If you have body-fat accumulation, especially around the waist and midsection (i.e., belly fat), it suggests that your liver may not be functioning properly or as efficiently as it could. To lose this excess weight, you have to detoxify and cleanse the liver, which leads to not only a slimmer waistline but also a thinner body.

The most common liver disease in America is a condition known as fatty liver disease, in which the liver stops processing fat and begins storing it right around the waistline. The main characteristic of fatty liver disease is too much fat stored in liver cells. In the United States, fatty liver disease affects eighty to one hundred million adults. The major cause of fatty liver disease is overconsumption of sugar, high-fructose corn syrup, and refined carbohydrates (such as white flour, white rice, and white sugar).

Our skin, sleep, moods, energy, and longevity all depend on the liver's ability to function optimally. The great news is that the liver is resilient and can easily regenerate itself. Even if a piece of the liver is cut off, the organ will regrow and continue to function.

As I advised in my book *Green Smoothies for Life*, one easy way to cleanse the liver is to take herbs or supplements, such as milk thistle, dandelion root, and burdock. These herbs are all-natural and very effective at liver detoxification. You will find that many products on the market combine these herbs into one supplement so that you can achieve the best results. As you look for products to help you cleanse your liver, be sure to use only those that are all-natural and gentle on the body. My favorite liver supplement is one I created called Liver Focus, which can be found on JJSmithOnline.com.

Additionally, an inexpensive liver-cleansing option is to drink one to two tablespoons of apple cider vinegar in eight ounces of water every morning and night. Do this for two to three weeks, or until your sluggish-liver symptoms have improved. Although the supplement is more potent and effective, drinking apple cider vinegar is a less costly alternative. It is fine to use ACV as a liver cleanse as just described, while completing the 7-Day ACV Cleanse.

Follow a liver-cleansing routine for a few weeks to a few months until fat burning increases in the body. Additionally, you may notice that the symptoms of a sluggish liver improve.

Symptoms of a sluggish liver include:

- Belly fat or fat around the abdomen
- Sclera (white part of the eye) no longer white
- Poor skin tone, including acne or breakouts around the nose, cheeks, and chin
- Dark circles under the eyes
- Yellow-coated tongue
- Bitter taste in the mouth
- Headaches
- Moodiness and irritability

Completing a liver cleanse can be a positive and rejuvenating experience that yields numerous health benefits. As you improve your liver health, you increase your body's ability to detoxify itself, expand its fat-burning capabilities, and achieve optimum overall health.

Digestive Cleansing

Periodic digestive cleansing clears the colon by removing waste that may be stuck along the colon walls. This excess waste can produce toxins that enter the bloodstream, causing various symptoms ranging from bloating, gas, and fatigue to acne and belly fat.

One way to cleanse the colon is with herbs and supplements taken in the form of powders or capsules. These treatments can help it expel its contents and draw out old fecal matter. You can find colon-cleansing supplements online or in health food stores, supermarkets, and drugstores.

One of the main theories behind colon cleansing is that undigested foods can cause mucus buildup in the colon. This buildup produces toxins, which enter the bloodstream, circulating and poisoning the body. Thus colon cleansing will clear toxins from the body or neutralize them and will eliminate excess mucus and congestion.

A nice benefit of digestive cleansing is the reduction of constipation. A poor diet that deprives you of essential nutrients can cause a plaque-like substance to form along the intestinal walls. Digestive cleansing not only helps remove the junk from intestinal walls, it also allows waste to pass more freely. The other noticeable benefit is the elimination of diarrhea, which is normally caused by toxins and can trigger problems for the whole process of solidifying the waste.

Look at Your Poop

A good way to evaluate your health is to check your poop. Bowel movements (BMs) that are black or reddish indicate potential health problems. Thin BMs suggest that your diet needs more fiber or that there is some type of imbalance in the digestive tract. If you have chronic constipation and your BMs are rock-solid, this may be an indication that your liver is overworked.

If you experience chronic constipation or difficult bowel movements for an extended period, you should seek medical advice.

Your bowel movements will help you understand what is going on with your body. Healthy bowel movements:

- Should occur one to three times a day, definitely no less than once per day
- Should not have a strong, foul odor
- Should be medium brown in color, shaped like a banana, and about the width of a sausage
- Should float, not sink to the bottom of the toilet

A very powerful and effective digestive cleanser that I have used for overnight results is a magnesium-oxygen supplement. It combines magnesium oxide compounds that have been ozonated and stabilized to release oxygen throughout the entire digestive system for twelve hours or more. The magnesium acts as a vehicle to transport oxygen throughout the body and has the gentle effect of loosening toxins and acidic waste as it transports them out of the body. Oxygen also supports the growth of friendly bacteria that are essential for proper digestive and intestinal health.

Magnesium-oxygen supplements are safe for regular use, but I would recommend they be used sparingly during heavy detoxification and fasting periods to help keep the colon clean and increase bowel activity. My favorite brand is Mag O7, which has been helpful in my personal journey of cleansing and detoxification. While using Mag O7, some clients have experienced decreased bloating, gas, and constipation. However, for me, it's knowing that I am eliminating toxins and waste from my entire digestive tract that provides the biggest benefit.

For intensive digestive cleansing, magnesium-oxygen supplements taken for seven to ten days are an effective way to jump-start any weight-loss program. They are safe for regular use and can also be used on a longer-term basis for daily, ongoing detoxification. In contrast to laxatives like senna, a high-quality magnesium-oxygen supplement is non-habit-forming and actually strengthens all organ functions, making it a safe long-term option.

As always, check with your doctor, and be sure to follow the directions on the product label. For most people, anywhere from three to five supplements taken at bedtime for seven to ten days will provide an effective digestive cleansing. If you experience loose stools or other side effects, simply reduce the dosage and be sure to take the supplement just once a day. Remember to watch the stool to see what comes out. You will be amazed, and possibly disgusted.

Coffee and Green Tea

Drinking one cup of coffee or green tea per day while on the program is recommended because these drinks contain very few calories and won't derail your weight loss. While you cannot add sugar, cream, or milk to your coffee or tea, you can add stevia or a nondairy creamer. Of course, you can also drink it plain. Be careful of the coffee and green tea beverages in coffee shops because most contain added sugars, syrups, or dairy products.

Green tea has tremendous health benefits and is particularly helpful in reducing body fat and weight, stimulating digestion, and preventing high blood pressure. Research shows it to be twenty times more effective in slowing the aging process than vitamin E because of its strong antioxidant capacity. The vitamin C content of green tea is four times higher than that of lemon juice. There are many wonderful benefits of drinking green tea, but as far as weight loss goes, it simply helps the body burn fat faster and more efficiently.

Green tea is actually better than black tea or coffee because its caffeine works in a different way. Green tea makes the body's own energy use more efficient, thereby improving vitality and stamina without the up-and-down effect typically experienced with caffeine. This is due to the large amounts of tannins in green tea that ensure the caffeine travels to the brain in small quantities, which harmonizes the energies in the body.

Just a quick note about caffeine: About half the research shows caffeine from coffee and tea to be beneficial, and about half suggests it has detrimental effects on the body. I am with the half that says it can be beneficial and can improve the fat-burning process. Therefore I recommend consuming some caffeine drinks—such as green tea or coffee—in moderation during this program.

Fiber

What is fiber? Fiber is the indigestible part of fruits, seeds, vegetables, whole grains, and other edible plants. Eating more fiber will help push toxins out of the body and into your toilet bowl via bowel movements. By eating more fiber, you strengthen the body's natural detoxification systems.

We take in environmental toxins (e.g., pesticides and herbicides) every day, and over time some of them stick to the colon and intestines in the body. This can prevent essential nutrients from being absorbed as well as cause weight gain and bloating. When we consume extra fiber, it attaches to the toxins and pulls them out of the body through our bowel movements. If you don't consume enough fiber in your diet, the toxins can remain in your colon too long and be reabsorbed into the body. By eating more fiber every day, you help prevent this toxic buildup.

Additionally, if you are trying to lose weight, fiber is known as a miracle nutrient that helps to regulate blood sugar, control hunger, and increase the feeling of fullness (satiety), which will help you lose pounds and maintain your ideal weight for a lifetime.

Processed foods and refined sugars in our diet have taken the place of fiber-rich fruits and vegetables, leaving us vulnerable to poor health and weight gain. However, eating about 30 grams of fiber per day will help you lose weight, prevent disease, and achieve optimum health. Fiber is a natural appetite suppressant: it curbs your appetite so that you can more easily reduce your caloric intake. Fiber will also improve your digestion and help you maintain bowel regularity.

According to Brenda Watson, author of *The Fiber35 Diet: Nature's Weight Loss Secret*, for every gram of fiber you eat, you can potentially eliminate 7 calories. This means that if you consume 35 grams of fiber daily, you will burn 245 extra calories a day.

There are two basic types of fiber: soluble and insoluble.

Soluble fiber dissolves and breaks down in water, forming a thick gel. Some food sources of soluble fiber include apples, oranges, peaches, nuts, barley, beets, carrots, cranberries, lentils, oats, and peas. Soluble fiber slows the absorption of food after meals and thus helps regulate blood sugar and insulin levels, reducing fat storage in the body. It also removes unwanted toxins, lowers cholesterol, and reduces the risk of heart disease and gallstones.

Insoluble fiber (also known as roughage) does not dissolve in water or break down in your digestive system. Insoluble fiber passes through the gastrointestinal tract almost intact. Some food sources of insoluble fiber include green leafy vegetables, seeds and nuts, fruit skins, potato skins, vegetable skins, wheat bran, and whole grains. Insoluble fiber not only promotes weight loss and relieves constipation, it also assists in the removal of cancer-causing substances from the colon wall. It helps to prevent the formation of gallstones by binding with bile acids and removing cholesterol before stones can form; thus ingestion of this type of fiber is especially beneficial to people with diabetes or colon cancer.

You will want to consume both soluble and insoluble fiber because each type provides benefits to the body. Many health organizations recommend that people consume 20 to 35 grams of fiber per day, not to exceed 50 grams. To support weight-loss efforts and improve colon and digestive health, I recommend a fiber intake of a minimum of 30 grams per day. The average American consumes only 10 to 15 grams of fiber daily.

If you're increasing your fiber intake, it is important to drink plenty of water to avoid constipation. Again, as I've emphasized elsewhere in this book, a good rule of thumb is to drink half your body weight in ounces of water daily. To determine how much this is, just divide your body weight (in pounds) by two and drink that number of ounces of water per day. So if you weigh 140 pounds, say, then you want to drink seventy ounces (about nine 8-ounce glasses) of water daily.

Given that your daily calorie count is important during this program, I recommend you take a fiber supplement to get more fiber in your daily diet instead of eating more fiber-rich foods. Some of my favorite brands of fiber supplements include Heather's Tummy Fiber, Thorne FiberMend, and Fiber35 Diet Sprinkle Fiber.

chapter 6

30 Recipes for Continued Weight Loss after the 7-Day Apple Cider Vinegar Cleanse

Congratulations on completing the 7-Day Apple Cider Vinegar Cleanse and taking back control of your health and your weight. Your body will be slim, healthy, and vibrant! Now it is time to continue to a lifestyle of health and wellness. You have put in the work and your body is rewarding you for your efforts. So be steadfast in maintaining consistency and good eating habits. You are on your way to finally reaching your goal weight.

It is of utmost importance that you slowly begin adding whole foods back into your diet since you have not been eating your normal diet for a time and your body has been cleansing. You may feel tempted to eat a lot, but this can be very damaging to your system. Take at least a day to reintroduce whole foods into your diet.

The 7-Day ACV Cleanse gives you a jump-start of losing up to fifteen pounds, but you want to win for the long term. To ensure continued weight-loss success and a healthy lifestyle, follow the Intermittent Fasting protocol and these six guidelines:

1. *Do the 7-Day ACV Cleanse once a month:* To accelerate weight loss, you can repeat the cleanse once a month. I do not recommend that anyone stay on the ACV Cleanse for longer than seven days straight. You should always give your body a break after a detox cleanse or fast. This keeps your metabolism revved up by mixing the foods you eat each week.

2. *Enjoy a variety of drinks.* Drink at least eight glasses of water (sixty-four ounces) per day, and drink detox or herbal teas as desired. Ideally, you want to drink the detox tea first thing every morning, as it aids in the detox process by cleansing the detox organs—kidneys, liver, skin, etc. You can also enjoy one cup of coffee or green tea per day.

3. *Avoid unhealthy foods the majority of the time.* Do not eat any white sugar, red meat, cow's milk, liquor, beer, sodas/ diet sodas, processed foods, fried foods, or refined carbs (white bread, pastas, donuts, etc.). In this chapter, I have provided thirty healthy, clean recipes that you can savor to continue a healthy lifestyle.

4. *Get moving.* It is important to move at least three to four days per week. You can enjoy any type of physical activity

that meets your fitness level, even if it's just walking for twenty to thirty minutes. Exercise is great for overall health, and we should all do it! If you become more active, you will enhance both your weight-loss efforts and your overall health.

5. *Have one or two cheat meals per week.* Cheat meals are great for tricking your metabolism. To prevent your body from adapting to a certain number of calories or a certain amount of food it expects to receive, it's a good idea to vary how much food you eat from day to day and allow yourself a few cheat meals. By doing so, you keep your metabolism constantly guessing. A few times a week, consider eating more food or a heavier meal. Your metabolism will become more efficient as it stays in fat-burning mode.

6. *Have one optional splurge per week.* You can savor a special treat or dessert once a week while on this meal plan. To maximize weight loss, it's important to keep desserts to a minimum and not overindulge. Learn to make healthy, clean dessert choices.

The Detailed Recipes

The unifying theme for these recipes is the apple cider vinegar. They use ACV in varying degrees, since we've learned in this book that ACV is key to healthy weight loss, reduced appetite, and stable blood sugar levels. Additionally, most of these ACV recipes add the perfect acidic and tart taste to many of your favorite foods.

List of Thirty Recipes

1. Flavorful Fried Eggs
2. Overnight Apples and Oats
3. Turkey Sausage and Apple Sweet Potato Hash
4. Chicken Sausage Frittata
5. Crustless Veggie Quiche
6. Apple Pie Oatmeal
7. Chopped Salad with Tuna
8. Smoked Trout Apple Salad
9. Turkey Bacon Salad
10. Lemon Parmesan Zucchini Noodles
11. Cabbage Chicken Salad
12. Smoked Salmon and Pear Spinach Salad
13. Turkey Burger over Salad
14. Crab Caesar Salad
15. Veggie Gumbo
16. Spicy Lemon Chicken
17. Brown Rice Noodles and Chicken
18. Pan-Seared Steak with Corn Salsa
19. Walnut Apple Spinach Salad with Smoked Turkey
20. Flank Steak
21. Cod Seafood Packets
22. Almond-Crusted Catfish
23. Roasted Cilantro Shrimp
24. Balsamic Vinegar Halibut with Tomatoes

25. Filet Mignon with Herb Sauce
26. Spicy Peanut Dip for Vegetables
27. Baby Carrots with Green Goddess Dip
28. Zingy Chipotle White Bean Hummus
29. Crab, Beet, and Radish Slaw
30. Apple Crisp Vinegar Cooler

BREAKFAST

Flavorful Fried Eggs

MAKES 1 SERVING (CAN BE DOUBLED OR TRIPLED)

> 1 cup organic unfiltered apple cider vinegar with
>   the mother
> 4 large fresh thyme sprigs
> 2 medium garlic cloves, crushed
> 2 tablespoons olive oil
> 2 large eggs
> ⅛ teaspoon salt
> ¼ teaspoon ground black pepper

1. Mix the vinegar, thyme, and garlic in a small bowl or container. Cover and set aside at room temperature for at least 2 hours or overnight. Strain the vinegar into a glass jar or small container, and discard the garlic and thyme.
2. Warm the oil in a medium nonstick skillet over medium heat.

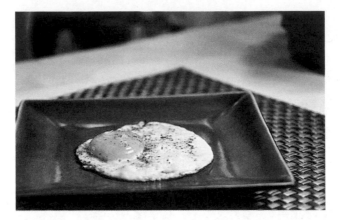

Crack an egg into a small custard cup or teacup, then slide it into the skillet. Do the same with the second egg. Season them with the salt and pepper.

3. Cook, undisturbed, for about 3 minutes, until the whites are set and the edges are browned and a little crisp. Slide the eggs from the skillet onto a serving plate. Top each with ½ tablespoon of the seasoned vinegar. Serve at once. (Reserve the remainder of the seasoned vinegar, covered and in the fridge, for salad dressings or more fried eggs for up to 1 month.)

Overnight Apples and Oats

SERVES 2

1¼ cups rolled oats (do not use steel cut or quick-cooking oats)

½ small sweet apple, such as a Gala, cored and chopped

1 cup unsweetened almond milk

½ cup organic unfiltered unsweetened apple cider

2 teaspoons organic unfiltered apple cider vinegar
  with the mother

¼ teaspoon vanilla extract

¼ teaspoon ground cinnamon

⅛ teaspoon salt

Stevia, to taste (optional)

Mix the oats, apple, almond milk, apple cider, vinegar, vanilla, cinnamon, and salt in a medium bowl or a 1-quart container. Add stevia to taste. Cover and refrigerate for at least 8 hours, or up to 12 hours. Serve cold.

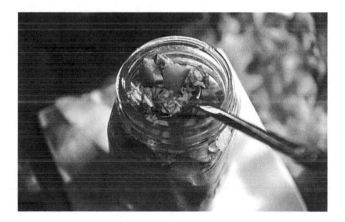

Turkey Sausage and Apple Sweet Potato Hash

SERVES 4

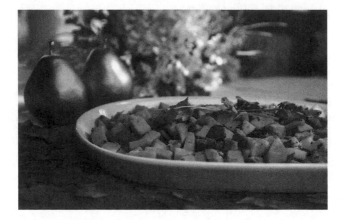

1 pound sweet potatoes, peeled and diced

1½ tablespoons olive oil

1 medium yellow onion, chopped (about 1 cup)

6 ounces turkey breakfast sausage, cut into 1-inch
pieces

1 moderately sweet red apple, such as a Gala, cored
and diced (do not peel)

1 tablespoon fresh rosemary, chopped

½ teaspoon salt

1 tablespoon organic unfiltered apple cider vinegar
with the mother

1. Place the sweet potatoes in a microwave-safe dish or glass pie
plate. Microwave on high for 5 minutes.

2. Meanwhile, warm the oil in a large nonstick skillet over medium heat. Add the onion and cook, stirring often, about 3 minutes, until softened and lightly browned.

3. Add the sausage and cook, stirring occasionally, about 3 minutes, until lightly browned.

4. Add the microwaved sweet potatoes, as well as the apple, rosemary, and salt. Arrange all the ingredients in one layer as evenly as you can. Cover the skillet and cook for 5 minutes to crisp.

5. Uncover and continue cooking for 5 minutes, stirring frequently, until the sweet potatoes are tender and the sausage is cooked through. Add the vinegar, stir well, and serve warm.

Chicken Sausage Frittata

SERVES 4

> 2 tablespoons olive oil
>
> 6 ounces sweet Italian chicken sausage, any casings removed
>
> 8 ounces brown button or baby portobello mushrooms, sliced
>
> 2 medium garlic cloves, minced (about 2 teaspoons)
>
> ½ teaspoon dried thyme
>
> Up to ½ teaspoon red pepper flakes
>
> ½ teaspoon salt
>
> 6 large eggs, whisked in a medium bowl until smooth

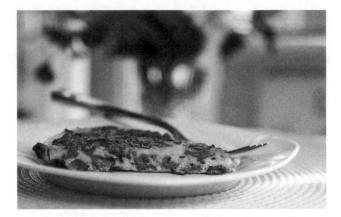

1. Warm the oil in a 10-inch nonstick skillet over medium heat. Crumble in the sausage and cook for 4 minutes, stirring frequently, or until the meat browns a little.

2. Add the mushrooms and cook for 5 minutes, stirring often, or until the mushrooms release their moisture and the skillet goes almost dry again.

3. Stir in the garlic, thyme, red pepper flakes, and salt. Reduce the heat to low and pour the eggs all around the skillet, not just in its center. Cover and cook for 10 minutes, until the top of the frittata is set.

4. Use a spatula to loosen the frittata from the edges and bottom of the pan. Slip it onto a cutting board and cut into quarters to serve.

Crustless Veggie Quiche

SERVES 4

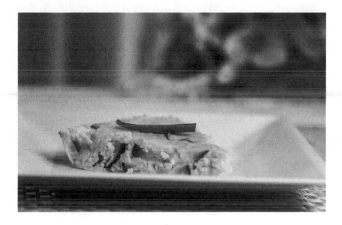

4 large eggs

½ cup finely grated Parmesan cheese

2 tablespoons olive oil

1 medium yellow onion, chopped (about 1 cup)

½ pound frozen cauliflower florets (about 2 cups; do
not thaw)

½ pound frozen sliced zucchini (about 2 cups; do
not thaw)

1 medium garlic clove, minced (about 1 teaspoon)

½ teaspoon salt

½ teaspoon ground black pepper

1. Position the rack in the center of the oven; preheat the oven to
375°F. Whisk the eggs and cheese in a medium bowl until well
blended. Set aside.

2. Warm the oil in an oven-safe, nonstick skillet over medium heat. Add the onion and cook, stirring often, for 5 minutes, or until very soft and lightly browned.

3. Add the cauliflower and zucchini. Cook, stirring often, for 4 minutes, or until thawed and thoroughly warmed up.

4. Stir in the garlic, salt, and pepper and cook until the garlic is fragrant, just a few seconds. Turn off the heat.

5. Whisk the egg mixture one more time, then pour it all over the skillet, not just in its center. Gently shake the skillet a couple of times to distribute the egg mixture evenly among the vegetables.

6. Slip the skillet into the oven and bake uncovered for about 15 minutes, until the eggs are set and the quiche is puffed up a bit. Serve warm.

Apple Pie Oatmeal

SERVES 4

> 5 cups unsweetened almond milk
>
> 1 cup steel cut oats (do not use regular rolled oats or quick-cooking oats)
>
> ½ cup chopped dried apples
>
> ¼ cup golden raisins
>
> 2 packets stevia
>
> Up to 1 teaspoon apple pie spice
>
> ¼ teaspoon salt
>
> Additional stevia, to taste (optional)

Mix the almond milk, oats, apples, raisins, stevia, apple pie spice, and salt in a 4-quart slow cooker. Cover and cook on low for 6 hours. The oatmeal can stay on the cooker's keep-warm setting for up to 3 hours. Add stevia to taste.

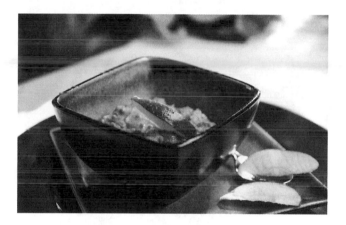

LUNCH/DINNER

Chopped Salad with Tuna

SERVES 2

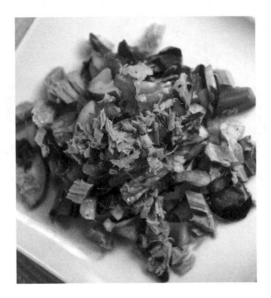

1 cup shredded, cored red cabbage

1 cup chopped, cored romaine or frisée lettuce

1 small green bell pepper, stemmed, cored, and
chopped

1 small cucumber, peeled, quartered lengthwise,
and chopped

1 medium globe tomato, chopped

3 tablespoons organic unfiltered apple cider vinegar
with the mother

2 tablespoons olive oil

½ teaspoon dried oregano

½ teaspoon salt

½ teaspoon ground black pepper

1 (6-ounce) can yellowfin tuna packed in olive oil,
   drained

1. Toss the cabbage, romaine, bell pepper, cucumber, tomato, vinegar, oil, oregano, salt, and black pepper in a large bowl.
2. Divide between two serving plates. Crumble half the tuna over each portion.

Smoked Trout Apple Salad

SERVES 2

2½ tablespoons organic unfiltered apple cider
   vinegar with the mother

2 tablespoons olive oil

1 teaspoon coarse grain mustard, preferably
   Dijon

1 small tart green apple, such as a Granny Smith,
   quartered, cored, and thinly sliced

½ small fennel bulb, cored, trimmed of stalks and
   fronds, and thinly sliced (optional)

6 large romaine lettuce leaves, thinly sliced

8 ounces smoked trout fillets, any skin removed

Ground black pepper, to taste

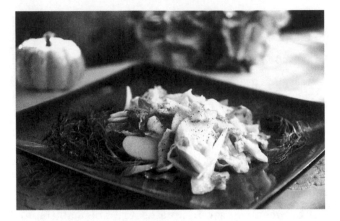

1. Whisk the vinegar, oil, and mustard in a large bowl until smooth. Add the apple, fennel (if using), and romaine. Toss well until the vegetables are evenly coated in the dressing.
2. Divide the salad between two serving plates. Crumble half the smoked trout over each salad. Season with pepper to taste.

Turkey Bacon Salad

SERVES 2

2 tablespoons plus 2 teaspoons olive oil

1 small red onion, halved and sliced into thin
half-moons

½ cup organic unfiltered apple cider vinegar with
the mother

4 cups chopped iceberg lettuce

4 slices uncured turkey bacon, chopped

½ teaspoon dried thyme

¼ teaspoon ground black pepper

1. Warm the 2 teaspoons oil in a small skillet over medium heat. Add the onion and cook, stirring occasionally, until softened, about 2 minutes.

2. Scrape the contents of the skillet into a small bowl. Cool for 10 minutes at room temperature, then stir in the vinegar. Set aside at room temperature for 1 hour. Do not clean the skillet.

3. Put the lettuce in a large bowl. Warm the 2 tablespoons oil in the same skillet over medium heat. Add the bacon and cook, stirring often, until crisp, about 3 minutes.

4. Scrape the contents of the skillet onto the lettuce. Use a slotted spoon to remove the onion from the vinegar and add it to the salad. Add 2 tablespoons of the seasoned vinegar from the onion, as well as the thyme and pepper. Toss well until the items in the salad are evenly distributed. Divide between two serving plates and serve warm.

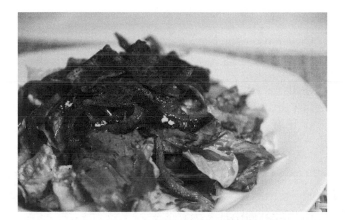

Lemon Parmesan Zucchini Noodles

SERVES 4

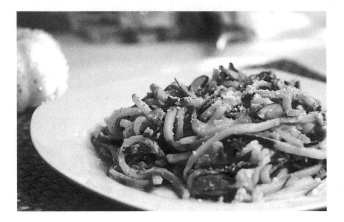

3 tablespoons sliced almonds

2 tablespoons olive oil

1½ pounds zucchini noodles

1½ tablespoons lemon juice

2 teaspoons fresh thyme leaves

½ teaspoon salt

½ teaspoon ground black pepper

½ cup finely grated Parmesan cheese

1. Dry-toast the almonds in a large nonstick skillet over medium-low heat for 3 minutes, stirring often, or until lightly browned and fragrant. Pour the almonds into a bowl and set aside.
2. Add the oil to the skillet, swirl it around to coat the bottom, then add the zucchini noodles. Cook, stirring constantly, for 2 minutes, until just wilted.

3. Add the lemon juice, thyme, salt, and pepper. Stir well. Then add the toasted almonds and the cheese. Toss lightly until well combined. Serve warm.

Cabbage Chicken Salad

SERVES 4

> 3 tablespoons low-sodium soy sauce
>
> 3 tablespoons plain (unseasoned) rice vinegar
>
> 1 tablespoon ginger juice (1 tablespoon of fresh grated ginger or 1 teaspoon of ground ginger may be substituted)
>
> 1 packet stevia
>
> 3 cups bagged shredded cabbage or coleslaw mix
>
> 1 large red bell pepper, stemmed, cored, and cut into very thin strips
>
> 6 ounces snow peas, cut into thin strips lengthwise
>
> ⅓ cup roasted unsalted peanuts
>
> 1 pound chicken tenders
>
> ½ teaspoon five-spice powder
>
> ½ teaspoon salt
>
> Olive oil cooking spray

1. Whisk the soy sauce, rice vinegar, ginger juice, and stevia in a large bowl until smooth. (*Note:* You can double these ingredients to make more sauce.)

2. Add the cabbage, bell pepper, snow peas, and peanuts. Toss until well coated.

3. Season the chicken tenders with the five-spice powder and the salt.

4. Lightly coat the inside of a nonstick skillet or grill pan with cooking spray. Set over medium heat for a minute or two, then add the chicken tenders. Cook for 4 minutes, turning once or twice, or until cooked through. Lay the chicken tenders on top of the salad and serve warm.

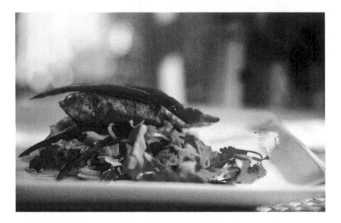

Smoked Salmon and Pear Spinach Salad

SERVES 4

½ cup chopped pecans

4 cups bagged baby spinach

2 tablespoons walnut oil

1 tablespoon no-sugar-added cranberry or
   raspberry vinegar
¼ teaspoon salt
¼ teaspoon ground black pepper
1 large ripe but firm pear, stemmed, cored, and
   cut into 8 wedges (do not peel)
8 (1-ounce) slices no-sugar-added smoked
   salmon

1. Dry-toast the pecans in a small skillet over medium-low heat for 2 minutes, stirring often, or just until very lightly browned and aromatic. Remove from the heat and set aside.
2. Toss the spinach, oil, vinegar, salt, and pepper in a large bowl until the leaves are coated. Divide among four serving plates.
3. Wrap each pear wedge with a slice of smoked salmon. Set two on top of each salad. Divide the nuts evenly among the four plates.

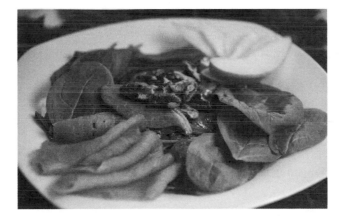

Turkey Burger over Salad

SERVES 4

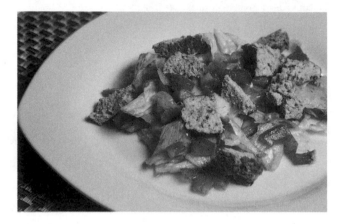

6 ounces white button mushrooms

1 pound ground skinless turkey breast

½ teaspoon dried sage

½ teaspoon dried thyme

½ teaspoon onion powder

½ teaspoon salt

½ teaspoon ground black pepper

Olive oil cooking spray

4 cups chopped, cored iceberg lettuce (about half a
    medium head)

1 medium globe tomato, chopped (about ⅔ cup)

1 small cucumber, peeled and chopped (about
    ½ cup)

1 small green bell pepper, stemmed, cored, and
    chopped (about ½ cup)

2 small celery ribs, thinly sliced (about ⅓ cup)

2½ tablespoons olive oil

2½ tablespoons red wine vinegar

½ teaspoon dried oregano

1. Place the mushrooms in a food processor, cover, and process until finely ground but not a paste.
2. Pour the mushrooms onto a triple thickness of paper towels. Gather the paper towels together to make a bundle, then squeeze most of the moisture out of the mushrooms over the sink.
3. Pour the mushrooms into a medium bowl. Add the turkey, sage, thyme, onion powder, ¼ teaspoon of the salt, and ¼ teaspoon of the black pepper. Mix until uniform. Form into 4 equal patties, each about ½ inch thick.
4. Lightly coat a large nonstick skillet with the cooking spray. Set over medium heat for a minute or two, then slip the patties into the skillet. Cook for 8 minutes, turning once, or until browned and cooked through.
5. Meanwhile, mix the lettuce, tomato, cucumber, bell pepper, celery, oil, vinegar, oregano, the remaining ¼ teaspoon salt, and the remaining ¼ teaspoon black pepper in a large bowl until uniform.
6. Divide the salad among four serving plates. Slice the turkey patty into small chunks and top each salad with the chunks.

Crab Caesar Salad

SERVES 4

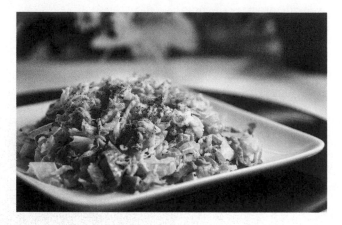

¼ cup sugar-free mayonnaise

2 tablespoons lemon juice

1 medium garlic clove, minced (about 1 teaspoon)

1 tinned or jarred anchovy fillet, minced

1 teaspoon crab-boil seasoning mix

4 cups chopped romaine lettuce

1 large green bell pepper, stemmed, cored, and
    chopped (about 1 cup)

2 medium celery ribs, thinly sliced (about ½ cup)

2 medium scallions, trimmed and thinly sliced

8 ounces lump crabmeat, picked over for shell and
    cartilage

½ teaspoon mild paprika

½ teaspoon ground black pepper

1. Whisk the mayonnaise, lemon juice, garlic, anchovy, and crab-boil seasoning in a large bowl until well blended.
2. Add the romaine, bell pepper, celery, and scallions. Toss well to coat. Divide among four serving plates.
3. Top each salad with a quarter of the crabmeat, then sprinkle with the paprika and black pepper. Add salt and additional pepper to taste.

Veggie Gumbo

SERVES 4

2 tablespoons peanut oil

½ medium yellow onion, chopped (about ½ cup)

2 medium celery ribs, thinly sliced (about ½ cup)

1 small green bell pepper, stemmed, cored, and
  chopped (about ½ cup)

1 (28-ounce) can no-salt-added diced tomatoes

3 cups no-salt-added vegetable broth

12 ounces frozen sliced okra (about 3 cups; do not thaw)

1 cup canned red beans, rinsed and drained

¼ cup green lentils or lentils du Puy

¼ cup raw buckwheat groats (do not use kasha, aka
  toasted buckwheat), quinoa, or millet

Up to 1½ tablespoons dry Cajun seasoning blend

2 teaspoons filé powder (optional)

Several dashes hot red pepper sauce, such as
  Tabasco, to taste

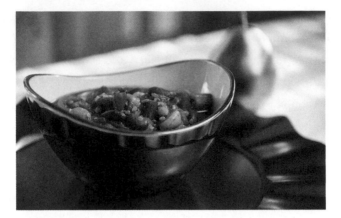

1. Warm the oil in a large Dutch oven over medium heat. Add the onion, celery, and bell pepper. Cook, stirring often, for 5 minutes, or until softened.

2. Pour in the tomatoes and broth; stir well. Add the okra, beans, lentils, buckwheat, Cajun seasoning, filé powder (if using), and hot red pepper sauce. Raise the heat to medium-high and bring to a boil, stirring quite often.

3. Cover, reduce the heat to low, and simmer for 1 hour, stirring occasionally, until the lentils and buckwheat are tender and the stew is slightly thickened.

Spicy Lemon Chicken

SERVES 4

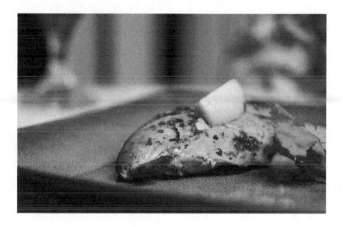

2 (1-pound) bone-in, skinless chicken breasts,
　　halved the short way

2 small lemons

2 tablespoons white balsamic vinegar

2 tablespoons olive oil

2 medium garlic cloves, minced (about 2 teaspoons)

6 fresh thyme sprigs

6 fresh oregano sprigs

½ teaspoon salt

Up to ½ teaspoon red pepper flakes

1. Place the chicken pieces in a one-gallon ziplock bag. Halve the lemons and squeeze the juice into the bag. Add the lemon halves to the bag as well.

2. Add the vinegar, oil, garlic, thyme, oregano, salt, and red pepper flakes. Seal the bag and massage the spices and juices all over the chicken through the plastic. Refrigerate for at least 1 hour.

3. Position the rack in the center of the oven; preheat the oven to 325°F.

4. Pour the contents of the bag into a 9-inch-square baking pan, arranging the chicken pieces bone side down. Bake for 30 minutes.

5. Remove the pan from the oven. Position the (hot!) rack about 6 inches from the broiler source. Heat the broiler. Return the baking pan to the oven and broil the chicken for 6 minutes, turning once, until golden and glazed. An instant-read meat thermometer inserted into the thickest part of the meat without touching bone should register 165°F.

Brown Rice Noodles and Chicken

SERVES 4

12 ounces thin brown rice noodles

¾ cup no-salt-added chicken broth

½ cup low-sodium soy sauce

¼ cup plain (unseasoned) rice vinegar

2 tablespoons lime juice

Up to 1 tablespoon hot red pepper sauce, such as
    Sriracha, Texas Pete, or Tabasco

2 packets stevia

2 tablespoons peanut oil

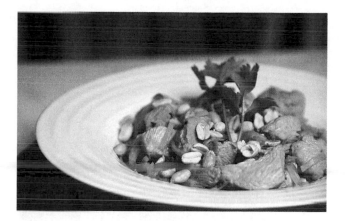

6 medium scallions, trimmed and thinly sliced

1 tablespoon minced fresh ginger

1 pound white-meat chicken cut for stir-fry (discard
any seasoning packet)

½ cup packed fresh basil leaves, chopped

¼ cup roasted unsalted peanuts

1. Put the rice noodles in a 13 x 9-inch baking dish. Cover them with very hot tap water. Set aside for 15 minutes.
2. Meanwhile, whisk the broth, soy sauce, vinegar, lime juice, hot red pepper sauce, and stevia in a medium bowl until smooth. Set aside.
3. Heat a large wok over medium-high heat. Add the oil, then the scallions and ginger. Stir-fry for 1 minute.
4. Add the chicken and stir-fry for 2 minutes, or until it loses its raw, pink color. Pour in the broth mixture and bring it to a boil, stirring occasionally.
5. Drain the noodles in a colander set in the sink. Add the noodles

to the wok and stir-fry for about 3 minutes, until about three-quarters of the liquid has been absorbed. Stir in the basil and peanuts just before serving.

Pan-Seared Steak with Corn Salsa

SERVES 4

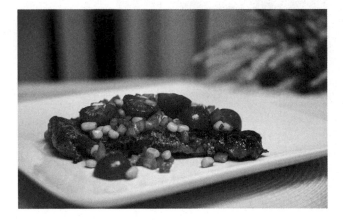

1 tablespoon olive oil

1 (12-ounce) boneless beef strip steak

½ teaspoon salt

½ teaspoon ground black pepper

½ small red onion, chopped (about ⅓ cup)

1 small green bell pepper, stemmed, cored, and
    chopped (about ½ cup)

1 cup corn kernels (if frozen, no need to thaw)

½ teaspoon ground cumin

½ teaspoon dried oregano

½ teaspoon mild smoked paprika

12 cherry tomatoes, halved

1. Position the rack in the center of the oven; preheat the oven to 400°F.
2. Set a large cast-iron skillet over high heat until smoking.
3. Rub the oil over the steak, then season it with salt and black pepper. Slip it into the skillet. Sear for 5 minutes untouched.
4. Turn the steak and put the skillet in the oven. Roast for 5 minutes, or until the steak is medium-rare.
5. Remove the (hot!) skillet from the oven. Transfer the steak to a cutting board and let rest. Set the skillet back over high heat. Add the onion and bell pepper and cook, stirring often, for 2 minutes, or until softened.
6. Add the corn, cumin, oregano, and paprika. Stir until fragrant, just a few seconds. Add the tomatoes and cook for 1 minute, stirring often, or until warmed through and a little softened (but not breaking down). Remove the skillet from the heat.
7. Slice the steak into thin strips and divide these among four serving plates. Divide the warm corn salsa among the plates, spooning it over the meat.

Walnut Apple Spinach Salad with Smoked Turkey

SERVES 4

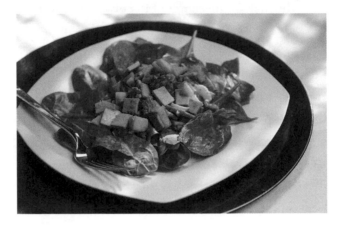

6 cups bagged baby spinach leaves

2 tablespoons olive oil

½ pound natural smoked turkey (no sugar added), diced

2 medium celery ribs, thinly sliced (about ½ cup)

1 large tart green apple, such as a Granny Smith, cored
and diced (do not peel)

½ cup chopped walnuts

2 tablespoons organic unfiltered apple cider vinegar
with the mother

2 teaspoons Dijon mustard

Ground black pepper, for garnish

1. Place the spinach in a large serving bowl.
2. Warm the oil in a large nonstick skillet over medium heat. Add

the turkey, celery, apple, and walnuts. Cook for 2 minutes, stirring often, until warm and fragrant.

3. Add the vinegar and mustard. Stir well to coat. Pour the contents of the skillet over the spinach leaves. Toss well to lightly wilt the spinach. Garnish each serving with pepper.

Flank Steak

SERVES 4

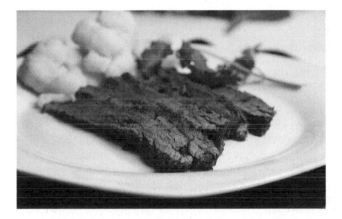

2 tablespoons olive oil

2 tablespoons chopped fresh sage leaves

1 tablespoon finely grated lemon zest

1 medium garlic clove, minced (about 1 teaspoon)

½ teaspoon salt

½ teaspoon ground black pepper

1 pound beef flank steak

1. Mix the oil, sage, lemon zest, garlic, salt, and pepper in a small bowl. Rub this mixture into both sides of the steak.

2. Set a nonstick grill pan over medium-high heat for a couple of minutes. Add the steak and cook for 10 minutes, turning once, or until medium-rare. Transfer to a cutting board.

3. Slice the steak into very thin strips and serve.

Cod Seafood Packets

SERVES 4

> 2 medium zucchini, diced
>
> ¼ cup sliced pitted green olives
>
> 2 (4-ounce) jars no-sugar-added marinated
>   artichoke hearts, drained
>
> 12 cherry tomatoes, halved
>
> 4 (4-ounce) skinless cod fillets
>
> 4 small rosemary sprigs
>
> 2 teaspoons dried Cajun spice blend

1. Position the rack in the center of the oven; preheat the oven to 400°F.

2. Mix the zucchini, olives, artichoke hearts, and tomatoes in a medium bowl.

3. Place a sheet of aluminum foil on your counter, then top with a sheet of parchment paper. Set a fish fillet and a rosemary sprig in the center of the parchment paper. Top with a quarter of the vegetable mixture and sprinkle with the Cajun spice blend. Fold

and crimp the parchment and foil together the long way, using the foil to make sure there are no gaps or holes in the seal. Then crimp and seal both ends of the packet tightly. Repeat this process, making three more packets.

4. Set the sealed packets on a large rimmed baking sheet. Bake for 20 minutes. Cool on the baking sheet for 5 minutes before opening and serving.

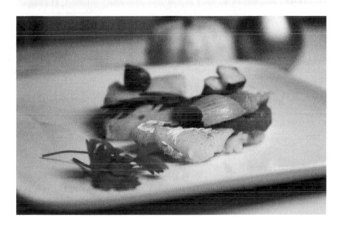

Almond-Crusted Catfish

SERVES 4

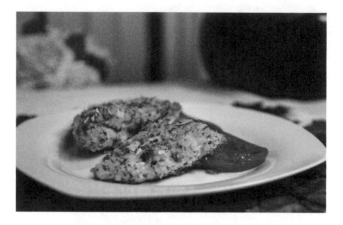

½ cup sliced almonds

½ cup whole wheat panko bread crumbs

2 teaspoons dried Italian seasoning blend

½ teaspoon salt

Olive oil cooking spray

1 pound skinless catfish fillets, cut into 4 pieces

4 medium globe tomatoes, thinly sliced

16 fresh basil leaves, rolled up together and then
     thinly sliced into shreds

1. Position the rack in the center of the oven; preheat the oven to
   375°F. Line a large rimmed baking sheet with parchment paper.
2. Mix the almonds, bread crumbs, Italian seasoning blend, and
   salt on a big dinner plate.
3. Spray the fish fillets with the cooking spray, then dredge them

in the almond mixture, coating them evenly and thoroughly on both sides. Set them on the prepared baking sheet.

4. Spray the tops of the fillets lightly with additional cooking spray, then bake for 25 minutes, or until browned and crunchy.

5. Arrange the tomato slices on four serving plates. Set a fish fillet on each, then sprinkle the plates with the basil.

Roasted Cilantro Shrimp

SERVES 4

> 10 medium tomatillos, husks removed and chopped
>
> 1 large yellow onion, chopped (about 1½ cups)
>
> 1 large green bell pepper, stemmed, cored, and
>> chopped (about 1 cup)
>
> 1 small fresh jalapeño, stemmed, seeded, and
>> chopped
>
> 2 tablespoons olive oil
>
> 2 medium garlic cloves, minced (about 2 teaspoons)
>
> ½ teaspoon ground cumin
>
> ¼ teaspoon salt
>
> 1 pound medium shrimp (about 30 per pound),
>> peeled and deveined
>
> ½ cup packed fresh cilantro leaves, chopped
>
> 1 small lime, cut into quarters

1. Position the rack in the center of the oven; preheat the oven to 375°F.

2. Toss the tomatillos, onion, bell pepper, jalapeño, oil, garlic, cumin, and salt in a large roasting pan. Roast for 25 minutes, stirring occasionally, or until the tomatillos have begun to break down and the sauce is bubbling.

3. Stir in the shrimp and cilantro. Roast for 7 minutes, or until the shrimp are pink and firm. Squeeze the lime quarters over the shrimp mixture, stir well, and serve warm.

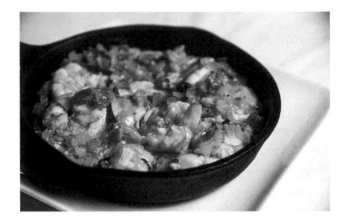

Balsamic Vinegar Halibut with Tomatoes

SERVES 4

4 (4-ounce) skinless halibut fillets

20 ounces grape tomatoes (about two 1-pint containers)

1 medium orange (for orange zest)

2 tablespoons olive oil

1 tablespoon minced fresh rosemary leaves

½ teaspoon salt

½ teaspoon ground black pepper

2 tablespoons balsamic vinegar

1. Position the rack in the center of the oven; preheat the oven to 375°F. Line a large rimmed baking sheet with parchment paper.

2. Place the fish fillets on the prepared baking sheet. Sprinkle the tomatoes around the fillets.

3. Grate the orange zest over everything using the large holes of a box grater. Drizzle the oil over the fish and tomatoes, then sprinkle them with the rosemary, salt, and pepper.

4. Bake for 15 minutes, or until the fish is firm and flakes when pricked with a fork. Drizzle the fish and tomatoes with the vinegar just before serving.

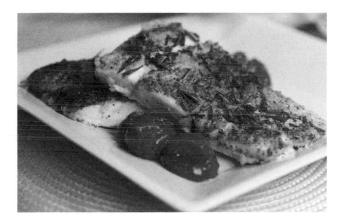

Filet Mignon with Herb Sauce

SERVES 2

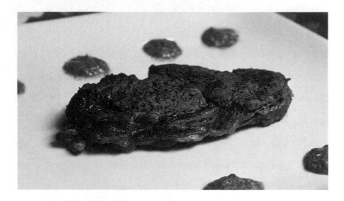

½ cup lightly packed fresh basil leaves

½ cup lightly packed baby arugula

3 tablespoons olive oil

2 tablespoons organic unfiltered apple cider vinegar
with the mother

1 tablespoon pine nuts or sliced almonds

1 medium garlic clove

½ teaspoon salt

Up to ¼ teaspoon red pepper flakes

Water as needed

Olive oil cooking spray

2 (6-ounce) filets mignons

½ teaspoon ground black pepper

1. Put the basil, arugula, oil, vinegar, pine nuts, garlic, ¼ teaspoon of the salt, and the red pepper flakes in a food processor. Cover

and process, adding water in 1-teaspoon increments, until the mixture forms a thick, spoon-able pesto sauce, stopping the machine once to scrape down the inside of the canister. Set aside.

2. Lightly coat a seasoned grill pan with the cooking spray. Set the pan over medium-high heat for several minutes. Season the filets mignons with the remaining ¼ teaspoon salt and the black pepper.

3. Set the steaks in the grill pan and cook for 5 to 6 minutes, turning once, for medium-rare. Dollop the sauce onto two serving plates. Set the steaks on top of the pesto.

SNACKS

Spicy Peanut Dip for Vegetables
SERVES 4 TO 6

> ¼ cup coconut milk
>
> ¼ cup low-sodium soy sauce
>
> 3 tablespoons organic unfiltered apple cider vinegar
>   with the mother
>
> 2 tablespoons minced fresh ginger
>
> ⅔ cup creamy natural-style unsalted peanut butter
>
> 1 tablespoon honey
>
> 2 teaspoons hot pepper sauce, such as Sriracha or Texas Pete
>
> 1 teaspoon minced garlic
>
> ½ teaspoon yellow curry powder

Place the coconut milk, soy sauce, vinegar, ginger, peanut butter, honey, hot pepper sauce, garlic, and curry powder in a blender. Cover and blend until smooth, stopping the machine once to scrape down the inside of the canister. Scrape the dip into a serving bowl. Serve at once or cover and refrigerate for up to 2 days.

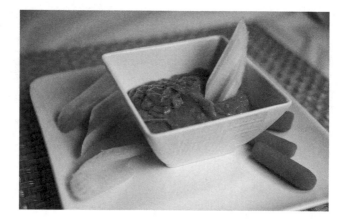

Baby Carrots with Green Goddess Dip

SERVES 4

   ¼ cup organic unfiltered apple cider vinegar with
      the mother

   ¼ cup olive oil

   2 large ripe Hass avocados, halved, pitted, and
      peeled

   ⅓ cup packed fresh basil leaves

⅓ cup packed fresh parsley leaves

1 medium garlic clove

2 teaspoons fresh lemon juice

1 teaspoon salt

½ teaspoon ground black pepper

1 pound baby carrots

1. Put the vinegar, oil, avocado halves, basil, parsley, garlic, lemon juice, salt, and pepper in a food processor. Cover and process until smooth, stopping the machine once to scrape down the inside of the canister.

2. Pour and scrape every drop of this dip into a medium bowl. Serve with the carrots. To store the dip, set a piece of plastic wrap directly against its surface in the bowl and refrigerate for up to 2 days. The wrap will stop the fresh herbs from turning brown.

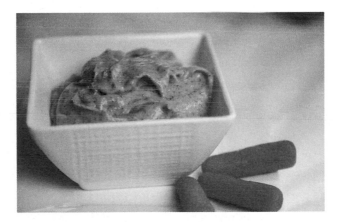

Zingy Chipotle White Bean Hummus

SERVES 4

1 (15-ounce) can cannellini beans, rinsed and drained

3 tablespoons organic unfiltered apple cider vinegar
with the mother

2 tablespoons tahini (sesame seed paste)

1 tablespoon minced, stemmed, and seeded canned
chipotle chile in adobo sauce

1 medium garlic clove

½ teaspoon salt

Put the beans, vinegar, tahini, chipotle, garlic, and salt in a food processor. Cover and process until smooth, stopping the machine once to scrape down the inside of the canister. If the hummus is too thick, add water in 1-tablespoon increments until the desired consistency.

Crab, Beet, and Radish Slaw

SERVES 4

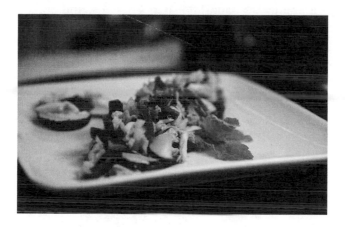

8 ounces cooked red or yellow beets

8 ounces large radishes

8 ounces crabmeat, picked over for shells and
   cartilage

6 tablespoons organic unfiltered apple cider vinegar
   with the mother

¼ cup loosely packed fresh mint leaves, chopped

1 tablespoon Asian fish sauce

1 tablespoon red hot pepper sauce, preferably
   Sriracha

1 teaspoon toasted sesame oil

1. Shred the beets and radishes with the shredding blade of a food
   processor or through the large holes of a box grater. You can also

get fancy and use a handheld julienne slicer to turn the vegetables into thin matchsticks.

2. Put the shredded vegetables in a large bowl. Add the crabmeat, vinegar, mint, fish sauce, hot pepper sauce, and oil. Toss well. Serve at once.

Apple Crisp Vinegar Cooler

SERVES 2

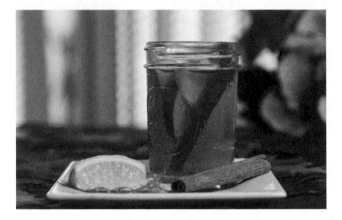

1 cup organic unfiltered, unsweetened apple cider

1 tablespoon organic unfiltered apple cider vinegar
with the mother

Ground ginger

4 drops vanilla extract

1 packet of stevia, to taste

Plain seltzer

Using two 12-ounce glasses, pour the following into each glass: ½ cup apple cider, ½ tablespoon ACV vinegar, a dash of ground ginger, 2 drops of vanilla, and ½ packet of stevia (or to taste). Stir, then top each glass with seltzer and stir again gently. Serve at once.

chapter 7

Frequently Asked Questions (FAQs)

Here are the most frequently asked questions about the 7-Day Apple Cider Vinegar Cleanse:

Can I use ACV pills instead of the ACV drinks?

Research shows that some manufacturers are able to convert unrefined ACV with traces of the mother into pill form. This means that the ACV pill can be a viable alternative to the drink. The ACV pills must be taken with a meal, not on an empty stomach. You will want to consume approximately 1000 mg per dose, which is equivalent to two tablespoons of the ACV liquid. There are numerous high-quality brands on the market, including NOW Foods.

How often can I do the 7-Day ACV Cleanse?

If you are overweight or obese, it is fine to complete the cleanse once a month. If you are at a normal weight but struggle with various health conditions, every other month is ideal. If you are healthy and at a good weight, once every three months is suggested.

How much weight will I lose on the ACV Cleanse, and will I regain the weight?

The amount one loses will vary by individual. However, most people will lose between five and fifteen pounds after seven days. If you follow the guidelines in chapter 4, you will be able to keep it off and continue on your health and weight-loss journey.

Is the ACV Cleanse similar to the ketogenic diet?

They are similar in that both will put the body into a metabolic state called ketosis. However, the keto diet focuses on a much lower carb intake. For example, the keto diet is typically 75 percent fat, 20 percent protein, and only 5 percent carbs, whereas the ACV Cleanse primarily emphasizes fasting (calorie reduction) and a diet of approximately 46 percent carbohydrates, 44 percent fat, and 10 percent protein. By prioritizing apple cider vinegar intake, the ACV Cleanse focuses on overall health benefits and not just fast weight loss.

Can I do just three or four days and get the same results?

The ACV Cleanse requires the full six-day regimen, with the seventh day being the transition day. Therefore we recommend following the program when you can complete all seven days, ideally Monday through Sunday.

Is there any online support offered while I'm on the ACV Cleanse?

We have a Facebook support group of more than a million followers that will encourage you on your weight-loss journey. You will need a Facebook account to join. We do the 7-Day ACV Cleanse as a group every other month. Go to: https://www.facebook.com /groups/Green.Smoothie.Cleanse.

If I don't eat all the foods on the daily menu, can I eat them the next day?

We do not advise doing so, as the foods designated for a single day should be consumed on that day in order to receive the proper nutrients. If you have leftovers, you can use them the next day, as long as you do not exceed the recommended daily calorie limit.

What if I'm hungry and need more food?

The daily menu should provide sufficient nutrients for your body. However, if you are feeling weak or light-headed, or having any other detox symptom, consuming another of the foods from the daily menu is preferable to consuming something outside of the diet. Additionally, if you weigh more than 250 pounds, it is okay to increase your calorie intake to as much as 1,400 calories on Days 1 and 2 and 1,000 calories on Days 3 to 6. If you need more calories/ food, be sure to consume what your body needs. However, the typical calorie intake listed for the program is simple and easy to follow for most people.

Does it matter which apple cider vinegar I buy?

It's best if you buy organic, raw, unfiltered apple cider vinegar with what's called the mother—strands of proteins, enzymes, and friendly bacteria that give the product a murky appearance and ensure that the nutritional benefits are intact. Bragg is a popular brand, though my favorite is White House.

Will I lose muscle during the 7-Day ACV Cleanse?

Many people think you lose muscle when you fast. This is not true for short-term fasting of four to six days. In fact, studies show a slight increase in muscle mass after a typical five-day fast. This is due to an increase in your growth hormone. You will not burn protein from muscle tissue until your body has run out of stored body fat.

Why is coffee allowed on the ACV Cleanse?

About half the research shows caffeine from coffee and tea to be beneficial, and about half suggests it has detrimental effects on the body. I agree with the half that says it can be beneficial and can improve the fat-burning process. One cup of coffee per day is fine on this program, but, of course, sugar cannot be used. Stevia is a great alternative.

Is there anyone who should not do the ACV Cleanse?

The following individuals should *not* do the ACV Cleanse:

- People over the age of seventy, unless they are in extremely good health
- People with any disease of the liver or kidney
- People who are underweight
- Anyone suffering from anorexia with an extremely low body mass index
- Athletes during competition or intense training sessions
- Pregnant women

The following people should do the ACV Cleanse only with their doctor's approval:

- People who take insulin or medications that lower blood sugar levels
- People with hypertension, cancer, or a cardiovascular, neurodegenerative, or autoimmune disease

What if I'm too challenged to make it the entire seven days?

If this seems like too big of a challenge, no worries. Always do the best you can, and be mindful that you're getting enough nutrients not to be *physically* hungry. You may be dealing with emotional hunger instead. You have to learn the difference between physical hunger and emotional hunger. If you feel the desire to eat even though you have eaten within the last two hours, you may actually be looking for a way to change your mood. Find something to occupy yourself for an hour or two. This will set your mind at ease. Then find a way to continually stay occupied or feel fulfilled until you eat again. I like to take walks, read books, and catch up with friends.

Should I take my medications during the cleanse?

I am not a medical doctor, so you should talk to your doctor prior to starting the ACV Cleanse. I personally would never stop taking any medications prescribed by a doctor. However, you must consult with your doctor, particularly if you take medications for diabetes, hypertension, cancer, or a cardiovascular, neurodegenerative, or autoimmune disease.

Are there any supplements that are important to take?

Certain supplements will ensure that you do not suffer from nutritional deficiency and will minimize detox symptoms. They include a mineral/electrolyte supplement, an omega-3 supplement, and a vitamin B complex.

What if I'm allergic to one of the foods on the daily menu?

If you are allergic to a food on the menu, replace this item with a different food from the daily meal plan. Be sure to match the calorie count so that you do not exceed your daily calorie limit.

Can I exercise while doing the ACV Cleanse?

Exercise is not recommended during the 7-Day ACV Cleanse. However, you may do light physical activity such as walking or yoga. Athletes participating in intense workouts or competition should avoid the cleanse altogether.

What if I am not hungry or don't feel like eating the food on the daily menu?

It is important to make sure your body stays hydrated and nourished. Try your best to eat all the food on the daily menu—this is not meant to be a starvation diet. The goal is to achieve a state of ketosis, and we do that by fasting with food.

How long can I stay on the full Apple Cider Vinegar Cleanse?

I do not recommend the ACV Cleanse more than once a month. Additionally, you should never exceed the seven days, as severe calorie restriction for extended periods of time will slow your metabolism and work against your weight-loss efforts.

What if my bowels are not moving?

As your body adjusts to the daily regimen of the ACV Cleanse, you may need help moving your bowels in the first few days. It is important to keep your bowels moving, ideally one to three times per day and never less than once a day.

If you haven't had a bowel movement in more than twenty-four hours, there are two methods to move your bowels.

Method 1: Use the saltwater flush, which involves drinking uniodized sea salt with water. To tolerate the taste, mix two teaspoons of sea salt into eight ounces of water; immediately after drinking this, follow with three more eight-ounce glasses of water. Do this first thing in the morning while you have an empty stomach, and you will have several bowel movements within thirty minutes to an hour.

Method 2: One product that works wonders at removing old fecal matter in your colon is Mag O7, which I highly recommend. Take three or four pills at bedtime, and you can look forward to a heavy bowel movement in the morning. Many of my clients use Mag O7 for regular colon cleansing.

chapter 8

Testimonials

I was so overwhelmed by the many testimonials from this 7-Day Apple Cider Vinegar Cleanse that I had to share. These are actual testimonials sent to me from those who completed the cleanse. My hope is that you will be inspired by their success and experience, and recognize that you can achieve similar results.

"I'm down 11 pounds! The success is giving me LIFE. I'm hollering, cheering, shedding tears of joy. I've had my oatmeal with berries and almonds this morning. Headed to brunch with family and have mentally prepared how I'll explain not eating or eating something super light."

—Kay T.

"I have lost 9 pounds and 3 inches off my waist. I am so proud of myself because I stuck with the ACV Cleanse. I made separate dinners for the family and didn't cheat one time. Now that I have seen results, I'm ready to continue."

—*Eileen C.*

"I'm so overjoyed with excitement! My clothes are sagging in areas, my mind is clear, energy is booming, and I look good!"

—*Quincy C.*

"Congratulations to everyone. I am down 15.6 pounds. My BMI went down from 42.8 percent to 39.7 percent. I actually look forward to exercising and hitting my goal weight."

—*Nicole T.*

"Ten pounds down! I'm so excited!"

—*Sandra B.*

"I'm so proud of myself! I'm down 9.8 pounds! I got a pep in my step and swag in my twist. I can't wait to see what the next phase brings. Thanks, JJ, for all you do!"

—*Faith A.*

"Oh my, I'm down 8.8 pounds in a week! My belly has gone down tremendously. On the morning of Day 5, I noticed that my thighs were slimming down because I was able to slide right into my pants without pulling and pulling like normal. I had no headaches or dizziness. I even took off work to focus on this cleanse without so many distractions."

—*Valerie B.*

"I lost 7 pounds but my waist is so much smaller. I'm only 5 pounds from my goal weight so this cleanse was just what I needed."

—*Carla D.*

"I'm so excited about what's happening with my weight. I'm down 7.8 pounds! My stomach and thighs are noticeably smaller. I'm excited to see the results in just 7 days. Hang in there, everyone. Thank you for sharing your knowledge with us, JJ!"

—*Tonia B.*

"I lost 5 pounds and a whopping 2 inches off my waist! I'm really proud of myself for sticking with it. I've gained so much discipline and self-control and realized food really does not run me."

—*Leela D.*

"I am totally proud of me. I am down 14 pounds! Feeling great and leveling up!"

—*Theresa R.*

"I am down 12.4 pounds this week. So proud because this week was the most stressful week I have had in a while, but I didn't fold. I can say, with my chin high, that I stayed the course and got my results."

—*Tammy K.*

"I lost 9 pounds based upon my scale at work. I am excited because I don't lose weight easily."

—Alicia C.

"I'm down 11 pounds. My stomach and face look noticeably smaller. I am winning! I didn't give in to temptation. #Proud."

—Alice B.

"I went from 170 to 162 pounds. I feel really great, thank you, JJ Smith!"

—Robyn J.

"I am down 6.8 pounds. It is not the weight that I lost that has me excited but the joy that I have gained in doing this cleanse. It has really given me new life. Thanks, JJ."

—Linda S.

"I am down 6 pounds, with a flatter belly, a ton of energy, and am now getting wonderful sleep!"

—Reesa K.

"I lost 7.2 pounds and inches as well. I didn't measure so I don't know how many but I can feel it. This is the first time in years that I'm totally committed to my health. I am so very proud of me. I so needed this!"

—Jen A.

"I am 10 pounds down and my belly has definitely shrunk! Now I have to stay the course and keep on track!"

—*Tamara B.*

"I'm so proud and happy to see my results. I am 10 pounds down and have lost several inches from my waistline. I love what I see. Thanks, JJ and team!"

—*Kelly T.*

"I lost 12 pounds and it feels good to lose weight again. I'm ready to continue this journey!"

—*Marlene B.*

"I am down exactly 14 pounds and I am truly ecstatic. I will continue this journey. I am ready for the next phase."

—*Lisa S.*

"I am down 8 pounds and have lost 4 inches off my waist in one week! I am feeling great!"

—*LaShawn D.*

"I am down 10.4 pounds! I will continue to have oatmeal and then head to the gym. I have to keep this going!"

—*Courtney N.*

"I am down 9.8 pounds in 7 days. JJ Smith has done it again. I feel great too!"

—*Deana T.*

"I'm feeling overjoyed. I released 10.8 pounds and 3 inches from my waist by following the guidelines set forth in the 7-Day ACV Cleanse. Losing the weight is wonderful, but the best part, for me, is that I now believe that I can accomplish my weight-loss goals. Both mental mastery and preparation were key to achieving my goals. Thank you, JJ Smith, for providing a blueprint for success."

—*Rachell L.*

"Tears came tumbling down. I lost 10 pounds in 7 days on the cleanse. I feel grateful and blessed."

—*Machelle M.*

". . . 10.2 pounds gone forever! I am so proud of myself! I even enjoy eating oatmeal now, when before I hated the texture. I feel great about these changes."

—*Cynthia L.*

"Life tried to get in my way but I had prepped and stuck to the plan. I have lost 7.6 pounds and 13.5 inches all over. This is in one week. I'm super excited to be able to go to the gym now. I want to see more and more results like this."

—*Brenda C.*

"I'm down 12.2 pounds in 7 days! Best of all, I finally broke through my plateau after 2 months. Thanks, JJ, for this well-put-together and easy-to-follow plan. Looking forward to more great results."

—Thea L.

"I am down 9.8 pounds. Thanks, JJ, for all you do. We did it together."

—Tamara W.

"I am down 8 pounds and 3 inches off my waistline. So motivated now. Very proud of myself."

—LaKesha M.

"I lost 9.5 pounds and 2 inches off my waistline. BAM! I will continue this journey because I am feeling great!"

—Patricia W.

"I lost 9.2 pounds. I'm so excited! Can't wait to get out of the two-hundreds. I am on my way. Almost there. Thanks, JJ."

—Crystal S.

"I am down 10.4 pounds. I cannot wait to continue this journey. My stomach looks remarkable. I'm not one who consistently gets on the scale but I feel lighter in the waist. I am constantly getting compliments at work."

—Gloria R.

"For a very long time I was stuck at the same weight. But I am proud to say that I am down 12.5 pounds. Thank you, JJ, you inspire us. The best part is more energy too."

—*Tamala R.*

"Unbelievable! Fourteen pounds gone forever! Two inches off my waist. JJ, I thank God for you, that you are using your talents and purpose in life to bless others. I am so happy!"

—*Chandra K.*

"Thirteen pounds gone! So proud of myself for staying on plan and finishing strong! I feel lighter in the body and mind!"

—*Gloria B.*

"I did it and I'm down 11 pounds. Living my best life. I notice a decrease in belly fat. I'm very proud of myself and the best is yet to come! Congrats, everyone!"

—*JoAnn C.*

"I am down 9 pounds and my clothes are no longer tight. I gained energy, confidence, and mental mastery! I even broke up with sugar! I lost all my unhealthy cravings for food. My appetite is suppressed! I am winning."

—*Kandi P.*

"I am down 13.4 pounds. My belly is starting to disappear and I still got to eat, I had great sleep too."

—*Pam O.*

"I lost 10.2 pounds while on my monthly cycle and I noticed that I didn't have any menstrual cramps. I'm sleeping way better. No cravings! I'm super excited so far."

—Lisa A.

"I'm down 12 pounds! Thanks for all of the support! I'm excited to finish this challenge strong! I'm back on track, no longer craving junk foods. Thanks, JJ."

—Bonnie L.

"I'm proud to report I'm down 15.4 pounds. It was very easy. I don't want to mess up my results so I am going to keep going."

—Janeen R.

"I'm down 12 pounds. I've lost the craving for unhealthy foods. I was able to get my mind right. Drinking water with lime and lemon helped a lot because I was able to flush my system out every day. I love having all this energy."

—Nicola L.

"I'm down 13.4 pounds. I thought my mind was playing tricks on me! I lost 3 inches off my waist. My energy and skin are on fleek! I wasn't even perfect but I finished strong."

—Elizabeth D.

"I am down 11 pounds. While on my cycle, I've felt no fibroid pressure as well. This is a bonus. I am very proud of myself."

—Alicia T.

"Congratulations, I am a winner! I stuck to the plan, did not deviate. I finished strong, 10.9 pounds down! Proud of my commitment, dedication, and focus. What a sweet, sweet journey. Excited about continuing to the next phase. Thank you, JJ and team!"

—*Laurie R.*

"I am down 12 pounds! I am so, so, so proud of myself! I truly changed my mind and relationship with food. I stuck with the plan as it was laid out. Thanks so much, team, for the support!"

—*Laney G.*

"I am down 8 pounds and 7 inches! I was hoping to see the scale budge a little more but I am pleased with my dedication and making it through the 7 days. Non-scale victories: better energy, clearer head/focus, and great sleep."

—*Avery B.*

"I finished and did better than expected. I am down 9 pounds, but more importantly, my blood pressure this morning was in the normal range. That's what I am working toward, being healthy."

—*Janeen K.*

"Congrats, sisters! You ladies are phenomenal! I lost 5 pounds. I'm at 149 now and my stomach is flat and I am seeing cuts in my stomach I never knew existed! My goal weight was 148, but now I want to get somewhere between 142 and 145. Happy Transition Day!"

—*Tammy S.*

"I just got on the scale. I am down 10 pounds and feeling good! I loved the ACV Cleanse because it helped me regain control of my late-night cravings."

—*Rochelle S.*

"I am down 7 pounds. I've also noticed that my waistline is shrinking. I'm even looking forward to starting new workouts this week. This program allowed me to focus on me and not the food. I didn't think this was possible because I love to eat. Let's go!"

—*Leah G.*

"I am so proud of myself and everyone else. Down 8.4 pounds, I am so happy and feel fantastic. I even took 2 inches off my waist and gained so much mental mastery. Thanks to everyone for their support. Y'all rock!"

—*Paula G.*

"I am proud of my mental mastery. I completed the 7 days even while traveling for work. I lost 7.2 pounds. When my family wanted to go to dinner, I ate my broccoli before we left so I wouldn't slip up. I have a made-up mind this year."

—*Monica P.*

"I lost 9.6 pounds and my knees and back feel great, not in much pain. I'm so proud of myself. This challenge made me feel brand-new and rejuvenated! Food is not controlling me. I am so excited. Thank you, JJ Smith, for giving us life."

—Cheryl R.

"I am so excited and feel great. I lost 7.8 pounds. I know my body is in the fat-burning mode! I feel great. All I can say is what the saints of God say . . . just keep letting the Lord use you, JJ! I know you were sent by God to help us break this weight bondage."

—Theresa H.

"Yes! Six pounds down but it's the inches I lost that I can't believe! I'm amazed by my upper body, arms, and legs are slimmer. Woop. Woop. Ready to finish strong."

—Lakeisha G.

"I'm glad I did the challenge and that I didn't substitute anything—10.2 pounds lost. I'm so ready and prepared for phase two. Thanks for all the encouragement through these 7 days!"

—Karen M.

"I am over the moon because I lost 3 inches off my waist and 8 pounds. Congrats to everyone on this journey."

—Tracy D.

"I am down 11 pounds. Any weight loss, inches, or clothes feeling looser is called winning! I feel amazing! So much energy! Let's do this."

—Monique R.

"I have lost 14 pounds, increased my energy, sleep better, and have the motivation I've never had before. I can't wait to see what's next!"

—Kim F.

"I lost 6.8 pounds and I lost 1 inch in my waist, belly, and hips. My bloating is completely gone, I am sleeping well, and my mental mastery has gone to another level! I needed this in my life."

—Naomi R.

"I'm not sure if this is normal but I am down 16 pounds. I guess I needed this in my life. I have never drunk so much water and tea in all my life. I'm loving my relationship with food right now. Also, my cravings are completely gone."

—Kira L.

"My jeans are swimming around my legs. I lost 7.2 pounds and 1.5 percent of body fat. Thanks, JJ, for all your guidance. You are a blessing. Showing us how to LOVE ourselves again."

—Laurie C.

"I am proud of myself; I am down 10.2 pounds in 7 days and lost 2 inches from my waist. My blood pressure is normal. I am so ready to continue this!"

—*Mary G.*

"I am 16 pounds down and have zero cravings for sweets. It's amazing! I feel great. I am so pleased with the results. Looking good again!"

—*Eloise D.*

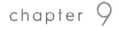
Using Apple Cider Vinegar for Home, Beauty, and Health

Apple cider vinegar has long been a classic home remedy because of its many benefits, ranging from soothing a sore throat to improving overall skin and hair health.

HEALTH

Weight Loss

Since apple cider vinegar lowers blood sugar and insulin levels, it can help with weight loss. The acetic acid in it helps to slow the absorption of sugar in the intestines. This will reduce blood sugar spikes that cause fat storage in the body. So ingesting ACV daily can be a useful tool in weight loss.

RECIPE: Combine 1 cup of water, 1 tablespoon of ACV, and 1 tablespoon of lemon juice. Drink this mixture up to three times daily prior to meals.

Liver Detox

The liver metabolizes fat and carbs and secretes bile to assist with digestion. This organ has critical functions for releasing toxins, digesting foods, and burning fats in the body. When your liver functions more efficiently, it is much easier for you to lose weight.

RECIPE: Combine 1 cup of water, ½ teaspoon of raw honey, and 1 tablespoon of apple cider vinegar. Drink this mixture up to three times a day.

Gallbladder Detox

The gallbladder is a small organ that holds a fluid called bile, which is secreted from the liver. Bile is the liquid that helps you digest fats and certain vitamins. The gallbladder works to remove toxins and to maintain the proper pH balance of the body. Maintaining the health of the gallbladder will provide long-term benefits.

RECIPE: Combine 1 cup of water, 2 tablespoons of organic unfiltered apple juice, and 1 tablespoon of apple cider vinegar. Drink this once per month.

Heartburn

With heartburn, the acid in your stomach travels up through your esophagus and irritates it, causing that burning, tight feeling in your chest. ACV is a moderate acid that brings down the pH level of your stomach acid and helps to relieve symptoms.

RECIPE: Combine 1 cup of water, 1 teaspoon of raw honey, and 1 tablespoon of ACV. Drink every 30 minutes until the heartburn symptoms subside.

Flatulence

There is nothing as uncomfortable or embarrassing as flatulence, also known as gas. Unhealthy foods will often wreak havoc on your digestive system. Even veggies and plant-based foods can cause excessive gas and bloating. The active acids in ACV can alleviate gas and reduce digestive distress.

RECIPE: Combine 1 cup of water, 1 teaspoon of peppermint extract, 1 teaspoon of raw honey, ½ teaspoon of cinnamon, and 1 tablespoon of ACV. Drink once a day, as needed.

Constipation

It is believed that ACV can alleviate constipation because it has large amounts of pectin, which is a soluble dietary fiber. Increasing fiber intake will typically ease constipation. The acidity of the vinegar can act as a natural laxative and will improve overall digestion.

RECIPE: Combine 2 cups of water and 2 tablespoons of ACV. Sip slowly.

High Cholesterol

Cholesterol is a fatlike substance that can build up in the arteries and cause them to narrow and harden, which places a strain on the heart because of the difficulty of pumping blood throughout the body. Apple cider vinegar can promote heart health by helping to reduce bad LDL cholesterol while increasing beneficial HDL cholesterol.

RECIPE: Combine 1 cup of water and 1 teaspoon of ACV. Drink twice a day.

Healthy Blood Sugar

Apple cider vinegar contains pectin, which slows the absorption of sugar in the intestines. Pectin helps you feel full and keeps you from having cravings between meals. ACV also provides enzymes that aid in digestion and help to maintain steady blood sugar.

RECIPE: Combine 1 cup of water and 1 tablespoon of ACV. Drink this mixture three times a day.

Yeast Infections

Apple cider vinegar has antifungal, antibacterial, and antiseptic qualities that will resolve the development of yeast overgrowth internally.

RECIPE: Combine 1 cup of water, ¼ cup of organic cranberry juice, and 1 tablespoon of ACV. Drink this mixture hourly until symptoms subside.

Asthma

ACV contains vitamin C and antioxidants that help to boost the immune system. When the immune system is stronger, asthma sufferers will have fewer attacks and can better stave off colds, respiratory infections, and environmental toxins.

RECIPE: Boil 4 cups of water with 1 cup of ACV. Inhale the steam from this mixture to open up airways to allow better breathing.

SKIN CARE/BEAUTY

Skin Toner

ACV is great for treating problems of the skin. It can be used to remove dead skin cells, cleanse the pores, and make skin appear clean and clear. ACV's vitamins and acids restore the natural pH of the skin as well, while removing dirt and oils from the pores, making them virtually invisible.

RECIPE: To make ACV skin toner, use a mixture of apple cider vinegar and water in a ratio that corresponds to your skin type. For example, if you have sensitive skin, combine 1 tablespoon of ACV with 4 tablespoons of water. You can use any unit of measurement—tablespoon, ½ cup, 1 cup, etc.—depending on how much skin toner you want to make at one time.

- Sensitive skin: 1:4
- Dry skin: 1:3
- Normal skin: 1:2
- Oily skin: 1:1

Dry Skin

Apple cider vinegar can bring moisturizing relief to dry, chapped, itchy skin and lips. ACV acts as a natural astringent to cleanse pores and remove dead skin cells to reveal fresh, new skin.

RECIPE: Combine 2 tablespoons of water, 2 tablespoons of witch hazel, 2 tablespoons of apple cider vinegar, and 2 tablespoons of castor oil in a covered container such as a jar. Shake thoroughly to mix. Use a cotton ball or cotton pad to dab the mixture on your skin wherever it is chapped and dry, including your face. Leave on for a few minutes, then rinse and continue with your normal skin-care routine.

Varicose Veins

ACV used as a topical treatment can help reduce inflammation of the skin and varicose veins and promote better blood flow and circulation. ACV has blood-improving qualities that will increase circulation and minimize circumstances that may aggravate the veins in the legs and feet.

RECIPE: Combine ½ cup of water and ½ cup of apple cider vinegar. Soak a washcloth with the concoction and apply directly to the varicose veins for 30 minutes at a time.

Acne

Apple cider vinegar can be used as a toner, facial cleanser, or mask to balance the pH of the skin to alleviate acne and other skin irritations. ACV's vitamins, minerals, enzymes, and acids work to regulate oil production that can help unclog pores that cause acne.

RECIPE: Combine ½ cup of water with ¼ cup of ACV. Apply to affected areas of the skin.

Hyperpigmentation

Hyperpigmentation is another name for dark spots, age spots, and spots caused by damaged or inflamed skin. This ACV mixture lightens dark or discolored spots, removes dead skin, and promotes skin-cell regeneration.

RECIPE: Combine ¼ cup of aloe vera gel, ½ teaspoon of ground turmeric, 1 teaspoon of vitamin E oil, 1 tablespoon of apple cider vinegar, and 2 to 3 drops of lemon oil. Mix well. Spread a layer on the face and neck, and allow the mask to dry. After 10 minutes, wash off with cool water and continue with your normal skin-care routine. Complete this regimen two to three times per week for desired results.

Sunburn

The most effective way to soothe and repair the skin after a sunburn is to apply natural healing elements that regenerate the skin's cells. The acids and enzymes in ACV restore the natural balance of the oils produced by the skin while alleviating the burning and tightening sensations caused by sunburn.

RECIPE: Combine ½ cup cool water with ½ cup apple cider vinegar. Apply directly to the skin with a sponge or moist towel.

Nail Fungus

Apple cider vinegar is effective in killing fungus and restoring nail health when it is applied directly to the areas where nail fungus is present. ACV naturally delivers antifungal properties that assist in the repair and health of nails and prevents future fungal growth.

RECIPE: Pour 1 cup of ACV into a bowl and soak nails in it for 20 to 30 minutes every few hours to kill nail fungus.

HAIR

Dandruff

Apple cider vinegar provides healthy acids that return the scalp's pH to a normal level by balancing the oils necessary to maintain moisture in the scalp. ACV can also improve circulation of the skin and reduce inflammation, resulting in a healthier scalp.

RECIPE: Combine 1 cup of warm coconut oil (liquid) with ½ cup of ACV. Apply to the scalp. Allow to sit on scalp for 45 minutes to an hour. Rinse out, then shampoo and condition hair as normal.

Split Ends

When the end of a hair strand breaks, it splits into two and continues to split the hair from the bottom up. ACV's vitamins and minerals provide immediate relief to split ends and help restore luster to the hair.

RECIPE: Combine ½ cup of water, ½ cup of mashed avocado, and ½ cup of apple cider vinegar. Rub on the hair, primarily the ends, and leave on for 30 minutes. Rinse and shampoo as usual. For best results, use twice a week.

Hair Growth

Apple cider vinegar stimulates blood circulation to the hair follicles, which is vital for hair growth and stopping hair loss in its tracks. Improved circulation allows blood to carry essential nutrients to the hair follicles for stronger roots and overall growth.

RECIPE: Combine ¼ cup of water, 1 cup of aloe juice, and 1 cup of ACV. Mix and apply directly to the scalp and hair, all the way to the ends. Cover with a shower cap and scarf and leave on overnight or for 6 to 8 hours. Rinse and shampoo normally in the morning.

Dry Hair

Apple cider vinegar should be part of your regular hair routine if you want moisturized, shiny, smooth hair. The acids in the ACV balance the pH levels in your hair and help to close the hair follicles, preventing dryness and split ends. This treatment will penetrate deep into the hair follicles and seal in hair moisture.

RECIPE: Place 3 tablespoons of coconut oil and 3 tablespoons of raw honey in a bowl and microwave for 10 to 15 seconds to melt. Then stir in 2 tablespoons of apple cider vinegar and 3 to 4 drops of lemon or lavender essential oil. Immediately rub the mixture into the hair, ensuring that all is covered from scalp to ends. Leave on for 10 to 15 minutes, then rinse and style hair as usual.

Product Residue

ACV is an effective treatment for ridding the hair of buildup from shampoos and conditioners. Clarifying enzymes and acids in apple cider vinegar act as a clarifier on the hair, easily removing residue left from various hair products.

RECIPE: Combine ¼ cup of water and 1 cup of ACV. Wet hair with the mixture from the scalp all the way to the ends. Cover with a shower cap and leave on for 30 to 45 minutes. Rinse and shampoo as normal.

COMMON AILMENTS

Sore Throat

Apple cider vinegar is acidic and can kill bacteria in the throat. It may also loosen irritating phlegm to relieve a sore throat.

RECIPE: Combine 1 cup of warm water, 1 teaspoon of raw honey, and 1 tablespoon of ACV. Gargle with the mixture or sip it slowly while it is still warm.

Cold and Flu

The acids in apple cider vinegar thin out mucus in the throat, allowing it to move out of the respiratory system more quickly, thus alleviating cold and flu symptoms. ACV also works to keep the body's pH levels balanced, boosting the immune system's ability to fight off infection.

RECIPE: Boil 2 cups of water, pour into a bowl, and mix in 3 tablespoons of fresh-squeezed lemon juice and 3 tablespoons of apple cider vinegar. Place your face over the bowl with a towel draped over your head to hold in the steam. Breathe in the steam for 8 to 10 minutes. Discontinue if it becomes too hot or you become uncomfortable.

Leg Cramps

Dehydration, nutrient deficiencies, and poor circulation can cause leg cramps. Potassium-rich apple cider vinegar will close this nutritional gap and reduce your risk of developing leg cramps, while also alleviating the associated pain.

RECIPE: Combine 2 cups of water and 1 tablespoon of ACV. Drink two to three times daily until symptoms diminish.

Insect Bites

Apple cider vinegar can hasten the healing of insect bites. The enzymes and acids even act as a deterrent to insect bites and stings, since bugs are repelled by the unappealing smell of ACV.

RECIPE: In a spray bottle, combine ¼ cup of water with 1 cup of apple cider vinegar. Spray the mixture onto the insect bite or apply to the affected skin with a towel.

Earaches

Apple cider vinegar's antiseptic and antibacterial properties make it effective in alleviating ear pain. ACV works to kill the infection and reduce pain and inflammation, easing the earache symptoms.

RECIPE: Combine ⅛ cup warm water with ¼ cup ACV. Use a dropper to drop the solution into your ear gradually over the course of 10 minutes. After 10 minutes, allow it to seep out slowly. Use hourly as often as needed, until symptoms subside.

HOUSEHOLD

Stain Remover

Apple cider vinegar will remove stains, lint, and grime from clothes.

RECIPE: Combine 1 tablespoon of apple cider vinegar and 1 tablespoon of white vinegar. Apply to the stain on clothing and let sit for a few minutes, then immediately wash the item normally.

Fruit and Vegetable Wash

Soaking fruits and vegetables in apple cider vinegar and water can reduce bacteria and pathogens; it will kill any fungus that may be present. The soaking will also extend the life of the produce.

RECIPE: Combine water and ACV in a ratio of 3:1—for example, 3 cups of water and 1 cup of ACV. Soak fruits or veggies in the solution for 10 to 15 minutes, then rinse.

Weed Killer

You can use apple cider vinegar to kill problematic weeds.

RECIPE: Combine 1 gallon of ACV with 1 ounce of orange oil and 1 teaspoon of liquid soap. Shake well. Fill a spray bottle and keep it handy to spot-spray troublesome weeds in your garden.

Unclogging Drains

Many over-the-counter drain cleaners contain toxins that can cause you to experience respiratory difficulties. Using ACV is a natural solution to unclog drains.

RECIPE: Sprinkle ½ cup of baking soda into your drain, then follow with 1 cup of apple cider vinegar. It will foam. After a few minutes, flush the drain with hot water. After 5 minutes, flush the drain again with cold water.

Wood Polish

Apple cider vinegar can be used to clean and polish wood furniture and other hard surfaces. It is also helpful in removing water stains.

RECIPE: Combine ½ cup of ACV with ½ cup of vegetable oil. Use a cloth or paper towel to polish wood furniture and other surfaces with the mixture.

chapter 10

Conclusion

Now that you've completed the 7-Day Apple Cider Vinegar Cleanse, you should feel accomplished, healthier, and lighter! Remember that I asked you to take photos and measurements? Well, it's time to evaluate how you did. Examine the photos for evidence of the subtle changes in your skin, hair, and vibrancy so you maintain the motivation to continue.

The body is fully capable of healing, rejuvenating, and restoring itself to optimum health. After these seven days, you will experience great health benefits. You will naturally slim down, think more clearly, feel energized, and notice improvements to your complexion as well. You will feel strong, empowered, and balanced.

I encourage you to live life the way it was meant to be lived: get engaged and be a full participant. Get out of your chair, get on your feet, and go live life. By following this program, you can achieve optimal health. You will enjoy your new body, energy, and well-being. It's time to get excited about your new life! It is not just about weight loss—it is a journey toward optimal health and wellness. You'll love the way your body transforms, and you'll be thrilled about your results.

If you prepare your mind and absorb the knowledge offered to you in this book, you will have all the power you need to become your best self and transform your life in every way.

Remember that you can continue doing the 7-Day Apple Cider Vinegar Cleanse every month to maintain the following benefits:

- Rapid fat loss, both total body fat and body mass index
- Decreased belly fat
- Improved dating and social life because of your slimmer, sexy body
- More energy upon waking, clearer thinking, and more productive days
- Ability to stay youthful well beyond what is typically expected
- Decreased blood sugar, contributing to the reversal of diabetes and a lower risk of insulin resistance
- Reduced inflammation, thanks to a decrease in several inflammatory markers
- Lower blood pressure and improved heart health
- Lower cholesterol levels, as you consume more foods high in heart-healthy fats

Are You Living Your Best Life?

When you live your best life, you are hopeful, optimistic about your current circumstances and your future. You are energized, enthusiastic, and passionate about living. We often feel passionate about life when positive circumstances occur, such as marriage or going on vacation after months of overdrive. However, this state of passion and joy can exist beyond the moment. By prioritizing your health and wellness, you will move into an everlasting state of happiness and satisfaction.

It is a feeling sparked by being challenged, growing, and achieving your goals (reaching your goal weight or receiving a promotion, for instance). Think about it: When was the last time you really pushed yourself beyond your comfort level, beyond your current state of complacency, beyond your current skill level and abilities? To live your best life, you have to push yourself, especially at times when you don't feel motivated. Motivation stays with us when we are fully engaged or challenged beyond our current level in life.

Motivation can also become addictive once you taste success. Get a glimpse of your best life and all the benefits that come with it—I bet you'll want more.

The magic of living your best life is that you are excited about the future again; you see your life developing into something greater. You begin to step outside your comfort zone and stretch yourself. You refuse to be lazy and apathetic because you know that laziness and success cannot coexist. You are able to maintain a heightened level of energy and excitement every day, and life becomes magical.

You wake up knowing that today will be better than yesterday as you become more of who you were born to be. As you set your plan for the future, you must be strategic about the choices, habits, and disciplines you apply. I have to do this every single day, because I am determined to live my best life—and so can you!

In closing, I want to leave you with my *10 Commandments for Looking Young and Feeling Great,* which I always share at the end of my seminars and books.

1. *Thou shalt love thyself.* Self-love is essential to survival. There is no successful, authentic relationship with others without self-love. We cannot water the land from a dry well. Self-love is not selfish or self-indulgent. We have to take care of our needs first so we can give to others from abundance.

2. *Thou shalt take responsibility for thine own health and well-being.* If you want to be healthy, have more energy, and feel great, you must take the time to learn what is involved and apply it to your own life. You have to watch what goes into your mouth, how much exercise and physical activity you get, and what thoughts you're thinking throughout the day.

3. *Thou shalt sleep.* Sleep is the body's way of recharging the system. Sleep is the easiest yet most underrated activity for healing the body. Lack of sleep definitely saps your glow and instantly ages you, giving you puffy red eyes with dark circles under them.

4. *Thou shalt detoxify and cleanse the body.* Detoxifying the body means ridding it of poisons and toxins so that you can speed up weight loss and restore great health. A clean body is a beautiful body!

5. *Thou shalt remember that a healthy body is a sexy body.* Real women's bodies look beautiful! It's about getting healthy and having style and confidence and wearing clothes that match your body type.

6. *Thou shalt eat healthy, natural, whole foods.* Healthy eating can turn back the hands of time and return the body to a more youthful state. When you eat natural foods, you simply look and feel better. You keep the body clean at the cellular level and look radiant despite your age. Eating healthy should be part of your "beauty regimen."

7. *Thou shalt embrace healthy aging.* The goal is not to stop the aging process but to embrace it. Healthy aging is staying healthy as you age, looking and feeling great despite your age.

8. *Thou shalt commit to a lifestyle change.* Losing weight permanently requires a commitment to changes . . . in your thinking, your lifestyle, your mind-set. It requires gaining knowledge and making permanent changes in your life for the better!

9. *Thou shalt embrace the journey.* This is a journey that will change your life. It's not a diet but rather a lifestyle! Be kind and supportive to yourself. Learn to applaud yourself for the smallest accomplishment. And when you slip up sometimes, know that it is okay. It is called being human.

10. *Thou shalt live, love, and laugh.* Laughter is still good for the soul. Live your life with passion! Never give up on your dreams! And most importantly . . . love! Remember that love never fails!

Now that you have experienced the power of the 7-Day Apple Cider Vinegar Cleanse, be sure to share your success story with others and help them to reclaim their health and vitality.

About the Author

www.JJSmithOnline.com

JJ Smith is a number-one *New York Times* bestselling author, nutritionist and certified weight-loss expert, passionate relationship/life coach, and inspirational speaker. She has been featured on *The Steve Harvey Show, The Dr. Oz Show, The View, The Montel Williams Show, The Jamie Foxx Show,* and *The Michael Baisden Show.* JJ has made appearances on NBC, FOX, CBS, and CW Network television stations, as well as in the pages of *Glamour, Essence, Heart and Soul,* and *Ladies' Home Journal.* Since reclaiming her health, losing weight, and discovering a "second youth" in her forties, JJ has become the voice of inspiration to those who want to lose weight, be healthy, and get their sexy back! She provides lifestyle solutions for losing weight, getting healthy, looking younger, and improving your love life!

JJ has dedicated her life to the field of healthy eating and living. Her passion is to educate others and share with them the natural remedies to stay slim, restore health, and look and feel younger. JJ has studied many philosophies of natural healing and learned from some of the great teachers of our time. After studying and applying knowledge about how to heal the body and lose weight, JJ went on to receive several certifications—one as a certified nutritionist from the International Institute of Holistic Healing, and another as a certified weight-management specialist from the National Exercise and Sports Trainers Association (NESTA). She is also a member of the American Nutrition Association (ANA).

In her most recent book, *Think Yourself Thin*, JJ developed and tested the seven mental strategies required for permanent weight loss. JJ's *New York Times* bestseller *Green Smoothies for Life* teaches readers how to lose twenty pounds in thirty days by incorporating green smoothies, healthy meals, and desserts into their eating regimens and discovering a lifelong approach to eating. JJ's earlier *10-Day Green Smoothie Cleanse*, also a *New York Times* bestseller, provides a proven plan to safely and quickly detoxify the body, and jump-start weight loss. Most people who follow the plan strictly experience weight loss of up to fifteen pounds in only ten days.

JJ holds a BA in mathematics from Hampton University in Virginia. She continued her education by completing the Wharton Business School Executive Management Certificate program. She currently serves as vice president and partner of Intact Technology, an IT consulting firm in Greenbelt, Maryland. JJ was also the youngest African American to become a vice president at a Fortune 500 company. Her hobbies include reading, writing, and deejaying.

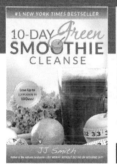
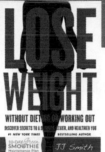
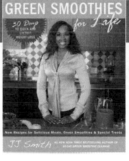
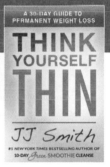